Eleven Blue Men

AND OTHER NARRATIVES OF MEDICAL DETECTION

Books by Berton Roueché

Black Weather

The Greener Grass

Eleven Blue Men
And Other Narratives of Medical Detection

Eleven Blue Men

AND OTHER NARRATIVES OF MEDICAL DETECTION

by

Berton Roueché

Do not fear to repeat what has already been said. Men need (the truth) dinned into their ears many times and from all sides. The first rumor makes them prick up their ears, the second registers, and the third enters.

— RENÉ THÉOPHILE HYACINTHE LAËNNEC (1781–1826)
REGIUS PROFESSOR OF MEDICINE, COLLEGE DE FRANCE

Little, Brown and Company · *Boston*

LIBRARY OF CONGRESS CATALOG CARD NO. 54-5121

Published February 1954
Reprinted March 1954 (twice)
Reprinted May 1954
Reprinted July 1954
Reprinted August 1955

Published simultaneously
in Canada by McClelland and Stewart Limited

PRINTED IN THE UNITED STATES OF AMERICA

The contents of this book first appeared in *The New Yorker.*

Contents

Eleven Blue Men

AND OTHER NARRATIVES
OF MEDICAL DETECTION

A Pig from Jersey

AMONG those who passed through the general clinic of Lenox Hill Hospital, at Seventy-sixth Street and Park Avenue, on Monday morning, April 6, 1942, was a forty-year-old Yorkville dishwasher whom I will call Herman Sauer. His complaint, like his occupation, was an undistinguished one. He had a stomach ache. The pain had seized him early Sunday evening, he told the examining physician, and although it was not unendurably severe, its persistence worried him. He added that he was diarrheic and somewhat nauseated. Also, his head hurt. The doctor took his temperature and the usual soundings. Neither disclosed any cause for alarm. Then he turned his attention to the manifest symptoms. The course of treatment he chose for their alleviation was unexceptionable. It consisted of a dose of bismuth subcarbonate, a word of dietetic advice, and an invitation to come back the next day if the trouble continued. Sauer went home under the comforting impression that he was suffering from nothing more serious than a touch of dyspepsia.

Sauer was worse in the morning. The pain had spread to his chest, and when he stood up, he felt dazed and dizzy. He did not, however, return to Lenox Hill. Instead, with the inconstancy of the ailing, he made his way to Metropolitan Hospital, on Welfare Island. He arrived there, shortly before noon, in such a state of confusion and collapse that a nurse had to assist him into the examining room. Half an hour later, having submitted to another potion of bismuth and what turned out to be an uninstructive blood count, he was admitted to a general ward for observation. During the afternoon, his temperature, which earlier had been, equivocally, normal, began to rise. When the resident physician reached him on his evening round, it was a trifle over a hundred and three. As is customary in all but the most crystalline cases, the doctor avoided a flat-footed diagnosis. In his record of the case, he suggested three compatible possibilities. One was aortitis, a heart condition caused by an inflammation of the great trunk artery. The others, both of which were inspired by an admission of intemperance that had been wrung from Sauer in the examining room, were cirrhosis of the liver and gastritis due to alcoholism. At the moment, the doctor indicated, the last appeared to be the most likely.

Gastritis, aortitis, and cirrhosis of the liver, like innumerable other ailments, can seldom be repulsed by specific medication, but time is frequently effective. Sauer responded to neither. His fever held and his symptoms multiplied. He itched all over, an edema sealed his eyes, his voice faded and failed, and the seething pains in his chest and abdomen advanced to his arms and legs. Toward the end of the week, he sank into a stony, comalike apathy. Confronted by this disturbing decline, the house physician reopened his mind and reconsidered the evidence. His adaptability was soon rewarded. He concluded that he was up against an acute and, to judge from his patient's progressive dilapidation, a peculiarly rapacious infection. It was an insinuating notion, but it had one awkward flaw. The white-blood-cell count is a reliable barometer of infection, and Sauer's count had been entirely normal. On Wednesday, April 15th, the doctor requested that another count be made. He did not question the accuracy of the original test, but the thought had occurred to him that it might have been made prematurely. The report from the laboratory was on his desk when he reached the hospital the following day. It more than confirmed his hunch. It also relieved him simultaneously of both uncertainty and hope. Sauer's white count was morbidly elevated by a preponderance of eosinophiles, a variety of cell that is produced by several potentially epidemic diseases but just one as formidably dishevelling as the case in question. The doctor put down the report and called the hospital superintendent's office. He asked the clerk who answered the phone to inform the Department of Health, to which the appearance of any disease of an epidemiological nature must be promptly communicated, that he had just uncovered a case of trichinosis.

The cause of trichinosis is a voracious endoparasitic worm, *Trichinella spiralis,* commonly called trichina, that lodges in the muscle fibres of an animal host. It enters the host by way of the alimentary canal, and in the intestine produces larvae that penetrate the intestinal walls to enter the blood stream. The worm is staggeringly prolific, and it has been known to remain alive, though quiescent, in the body of a surviving victim for thirty-one years. In general, the number of trichinae that succeed in reaching the muscle determines the severity of an attack. As such parasitic organisms go, adult trichinae are relatively large, the males averaging one-twentieth of an inch in length and the females about twice that. The larvae are less statuesque. Pathologists have found as many as twelve hundred of them encysted in a single gram of tissue. Numerous animals, ranging in size from the mole to the hippopotamus, are hospitable to the trichina, but it has a strong predilection for swine and man. Man's only important source of infection is pork. The disease is perpetuated in swine by the practice common among hog raisers of using garbage, some of which inevitably contains trichinous meat, for feed. Swine have a high degree of tolerance for the trichina, but man's resistive powers are feeble. In 1931, in Detroit, a man suffered a violent seizure of trichinosis as a result of merely eating a piece of bread buttered with a knife that had been used to slice an infested sausage. The hog from which the sausage was made had appeared to be in excellent health. Few acute afflictions are more painful than trichinosis, or more prolonged and debilitating. Its victims are occasionally prostrated for many months, and relapses after apparent recoveries are not uncommon. Its mortality rate is disconcertingly variable. It is usually around six per cent, but in some outbreaks nearly a third of those stricken have died, and the recovery of a patient from a full-scale attack is almost unheard of. Nobody is, or can be rendered, immune to trichinosis. Also, there is no specific cure. In the opinion of most investigators, it is far from likely that one will ever be found. They are persuaded that any therapeutic agent potent enough to kill a multitude of embedded trichinae would probably kill the patient, too.

Although medical science is unable to terminate, or even lessen the severity of, an assault of trichinosis, no disease is easier to dodge. There are several dependable means of evasion. Abstention from pork is, of course, one. It is also the most venerable, having been known, vigorously recommended, and widely practiced for at least three thousand years. Some authorities, in fact, regard the Mosaic proscription of pork as the pioneering step in the development of preventive medicine. However, since the middle of the nineteenth century, when the cause and nature of trichinosis were illuminated by Sir James Paget, Rudolf Virchow, Friedrich Albert von Zenker, and others, less ascetic safeguards have become available. The trichinae are rugged but not indestructible. It has been amply demonstrated that thorough cooking (until the meat is bone-white) will make even the wormiest pork harmless. So will refrigeration at a maximum temperature of five degrees for a minimum of twenty days. So, just as effectively, will certain scrupulous methods of salting, smoking, and pickling.

Despite this abundance of easily applied defensive techniques, the incidence of trichinosis has not greatly diminished over the globe in the past fifty or sixty years. In some countries, it has even increased. The United States is one of them. Many epidemiologists are convinced that this country now leads the world in trichinosis. It is, at any rate, a major health problem here. According to a compendium of recent autopsy studies, approximately one American in five has at some time or another had trichinosis, and it is probable that well over a million are afflicted with it every year. As a considerable source of misery, it ranks with tuberculosis, syphilis, and undulant fever. It will probably continue to be one for some time to come. Its spread is almost unimpeded. A few states, New York among them, have statutes prohibiting the feeding of uncooked garbage to swine, but nowhere is a very determined effort made at enforcement, and the Bureau of Animal Industry of the United States Department of Agriculture, although it assumes all pork to be trichinous until proved otherwise, requires packing houses to administer a prophylactic freeze to only those varieties of the meat — frankfurters, salami, prosciutto, and the like — that are often eaten raw. Moreover, not all processed pork comes under the jurisdiction of the Department. At least a third of it is processed under local ordinances in small, neighborhood abattoirs beyond the reach of the Bureau, or on farms. Nearly two per cent of the hogs slaughtered in the United States are trichinous.

Except for a brief period around the beginning of this century, when several European countries refused, because of its dubious nature, to import American pork, the adoption of a less porous system of control has never been seriously contemplated here. One reason is that it would run into money. Another is that, except by a few informed authorities, it has always been considered unnecessary. Trichinosis is generally believed to be a rarity. This view, though hallucinated, is not altogether without explanation. Outbreaks of trichinosis are seldom widely publicized. They are seldom even recognized. Trichinosis is the chameleon of diseases. Nearly all diseases are anonymous at onset, and many tend to resist identification until their grip is well established, but most can eventually be identified by patient scrutiny. Trichinosis is occasionally impervious to bedside detection at any stage. Even blood counts sometimes inexplicably fail to reveal its presence at any stage in its development. As a diagnostic deadfall, it is practically unique. The number and variety of ailments with which it is more or less commonly confused approach the encyclopedic. They include arthritis, acute alcoholism, conjunctivitis, food poisoning, lead poisoning, heart disease, laryngitis, mumps, asthma, rheumatism, rheumatic fever, rheumatic myocarditis, gout, tuberculosis, angioneurotic edema, dermatomyositis, frontal sinusitis, influenza, nephritis, peptic ulcer, appendicitis, cholecystitis, malaria, scarlet fever, typhoid fever, paratyphoid fever, undulant fever, encephalitis, gastroenteritis, intercostal neuritis, tetanus, pleurisy, colitis, meningitis, syphilis, typhus, and cholera. It has even been mistaken for beriberi. With all the rich inducements to error, a sound diagnosis of trichinosis is rarely made, and the diagnostician cannot always take much credit for it. Often, as at Metropolitan Hospital that April day in 1942, it is forced upon him.

The report of the arresting discovery at Metropolitan reached the Health Department on the morning of Friday, April 17th. Its form was conventional — a postcard bearing a scribbled name, address, and diagnosis — and it was handled with conventional dispatch. Within an hour. Dr. Morris Greenberg, who was then chief epidemiologist of the Bureau of Preventable Diseases and is now its director, had put one of his fleetest agents on the case, a field epidemiologist named Lawrence Levy. Ten minutes after receiving the assignment, Dr. Levy was on his way to the hospital, intent on tracking down the source of the infection, with the idea of alerting the physicians of other persons who might have contracted the disease along with Sauer. At eleven o'clock, Dr. Levy walked into the office of the medical superintendent at Metropolitan. His immediate objective was to satisfy himself that Sauer was indeed suffering from trichinosis. He was quickly convinced. The evidence of the eosinophile count was now supported in the record by more graphic proof. Sauer, the night before, had undergone a biopsy. A sliver of muscle had been taken from one of his legs and examined under a microscope. It teemed with *Trichinella spiralis*. On the basis of the sample, the record noted, the pathologist who made the test estimated the total infestation of trichinae at upward of twelve million. A count of over five million is almost invariably lethal. Dr. Levy returned the dossier to the file. Then, moving on to his more general objective, he had a word with the patient. He found him bemused but conscious. Sauer appeared at times to distantly comprehend what was said to him, but his replies were faint and rambling and mostly incoherent. At the end of five minutes, Dr. Levy gave up. He hadn't learned much, but he had learned something, and he didn't have the heart to go on with his questioning. It was just possible, he let himself hope, that he had the lead he needed. Sauer had mentioned the New York Labor Temple, a German-American meeting-and-banquet hall on East Eighty-fourth Street, and he had twice uttered the word "*Schlachtfest.*" A *Schlachtfest*, in Yorkville, the Doctor knew, is a pork feast.

Before leaving the hospital, Dr. Levy telephoned Dr. Greenberg and dutifully related what he had found out. It didn't take him long. Then he had a sandwich and a cup of coffee and headed for the Labor Temple, getting there at a little past one. It was, and is, a shabby yellow-brick building of six stories, a few doors west of Second Avenue, with a high, ornately balustraded stoop and a double basement. Engraved on the façade, just above the entrance, is a maxim: "Knowledge Is Power." In 1942, the Temple was owned and operated, on a non-profit basis, by the Workmen's Educational Association; it has since been acquired by private interests and is now given over to business and light manufacturing. A porter directed Dr. Levy to the manager's office, a cubicle at the end of a dim corridor flanked by meeting rooms. The manager was in, and, after a spasm of bewilderment, keenly coöperative. He brought out his records and gave Dr. Levy all the information he had. Sauer was known at the Temple. He had been employed there off and on for a year or more as a dishwasher and general kitchen helper, the manager related. He was one of a large group of lightly skilled wanderers from which the cook was accustomed to recruit a staff whenever the need arose. Sauer had last worked at the Temple on the nights of March 27th and 28th. On the latter, as it happened, the occasion was a *Schlachtfest*.

Dr. Levy, aware that the incubation period of trichinosis is usually from seven to fourteen days and that Sauer had presented himself at Lenox Hill on April 6th, motioned to the manager to continue. The *Schlachtfest* had been given by the Hindenburg Pleasure Society, an informal organization whose members and their wives gathered periodically at the Temple for an evening of singing and dancing and overeating. The arrangements for the party had been made by the secretary of the society — Felix Lindenhauser, a name which, like those of Sauer and the others I shall mention in connection with the *Schlachtfest*, is a fictitious one. Lindenhauser lived in St. George, on Staten Island. The manager's records did not indicate where the pork had been obtained. Probably, he said, it had been supplied by the society. That was frequently the case. The cook would know, but it was not yet time for him to come on duty. The implication of this statement was not lost on Dr. Levy. Then the cook, he asked, was well? The manager said that he appeared to be. Having absorbed this awkward piece of information, Dr. Levy inquired about the health of the others who had been employed in the kitchen on the night of March 28th. The manager didn't know. His records showed, however, that, like Sauer, none of them had worked at the Temple since that night. He pointed out that it was quite possible, of course, that they hadn't been asked to. Dr. Levy noted down their names — Rudolf Nath, Henry Kuhn, Frederick Kreisler, and William Ritter — and their addresses. Nath lived in Queens, Kreisler in Brooklyn, and Kuhn and Ritter in the Bronx. Then Dr. Levy settled back to await the arrival of the cook. The cook turned up at three, and he, too, was very coöperative. He was feeling fine, he said. He remembered the *Schlachtfest*. The pig, he recalled, had been provided by the society. Some of it had been ground up into sausage and baked. The rest had been roasted. All of it had been thoroughly cooked. He was certain of that. The sausage, for example, had been boiled for two hours before it was baked. He had eaten his share of both. He supposed that the rest of the help had, too, but there was no knowing. He had neither seen nor talked to any of them since the night of the feast. There had been no occasion to, he said.

Dr. Levy returned to his office, and sat there for a while in meditation. Presently, he put in a call to Felix Lindenhauser, the secretary of the society, at his home on Staten Island. Lindenhauser answered the telephone. Dr. Levy introduced himself and stated his problem. Lindenhauser was plainly flabbergasted. He said he was in excellent health, and had been for months. His wife, who had accompanied him to the *Schlachtfest*, was also in good health. He had heard of no illness in the society. He couldn't believe that there had been anything wrong with that pork. It had been delicious. The pig had been obtained by two members of the society, George Muller and Hans Breit, both of whom lived in the Bronx. They had bought it from a farmer of their acquaintance in New Jersey. Lindenhauser went on to say that there had been twenty-seven people at the feast, including himself and his wife. The names and addresses of the company were in his minute book. He fetched it to the phone and patiently read them off as Dr. Levy wrote them down. If he could be of any further help, he added as he prepared to hang up, just let him know, but he was convinced that Dr. Levy was wasting his time. At the moment, Dr. Levy was almost inclined to agree with him.

Dr. Levy spent an increasingly uneasy weekend. He was of two antagonistic minds. He refused to believe that Sauer's illness was not in some way related to the *Schlachtfest* of the Hindenburg Pleasure Society. On the other hand, it didn't seem possible that it was. Late Saturday afternoon, at his home, he received a call that increased his discouragement, if not his perplexity. It was from his office. Metropolitan Hospital had called to report that Herman Sauer was dead. Dr. Levy put down the receiver with the leaden realization that, good or bad, the *Schlachtfest* was now the only lead he would ever have.

On Monday, Dr. Levy buckled heavily down to the essential but unexhilarating task of determining the health of the twenty-seven men and women who had attended the *Schlachtfest*. Although his attitude was half-hearted, his procedure was methodical, unhurried, and objective. He called on and closely examined each of the guests, including the Lindenhausers, and from each procured a sample of blood for analysis in the Health Department laboratories. The job, necessarily involving a good deal of leg work and many evening visits, took him the better part of two weeks. He ended up, on April 30th, about equally reassured and stumped. His findings were provocative but contradictory. Of the twenty-seven who had feasted together on the night of March 28th, twenty-five were in what undeniably was their normal state of health. Two, just as surely, were not. The exceptions were George Muller and Hans Breit, the men who had provided the pig. Muller was at home and in bed, suffering sorely from what his family physician had uncertainly diagnosed as some sort of intestinal upheaval. Breit was in as bad a way, or worse, in Fordham Hospital. He had been admitted there for observation on April 10th. Several diagnoses had been suggested, including rheumatic myocarditis, pleurisy, and grippe, but none had been formally retained. The nature of the two men's trouble was no mystery to Dr. Levy. Both, as he was subsequently able to demonstrate, had trichinosis.

On Friday morning, May 1st, Dr. Levy returned to the Bronx for a more searching word with Muller. Owing to Muller's debilitated condition on the occasion of Dr. Levy's first visit, their talk had been brief and clinical in character. Muller, who was now up and shakily about, received him warmly. Since their meeting several days before, he said, he had been enlivening the tedious hours of illness with reflection. A question had occurred to him. Would it be possible, he inquired, to contract trichinosis from just a few nibbles of raw pork? It would, Dr. Levy told him. He also urged him to be more explicit. Thus encouraged, Muller displayed an unexpected gift for what appeared to be total recall. He leisurely recounted to Dr. Levy that he and Breit had bought the pig from a farmer who owned a place near Midvale, New Jersey. The farmer had killed and dressed the animal, and they had delivered the carcass to the Labor Temple kitchen on the evening of March 27th. That, however, had been only part of their job. Not wishing to trouble the cook and his helpers, who were otherwise occupied, Muller and Breit had then set about preparing the sausage for the feast. They were both experienced amateur sausage makers, he said, and explained the process — grinding, macerating, and seasoning — in laborious detail. Dr. Levy began to fidget. Naturally, Muller presently went on, they had been obliged to sample their work. There was no other way to make sure that the meat was properly seasoned. He had taken perhaps two or three little nibbles. Breit, who had a heartier taste for raw pork, had probably eaten a trifle more. It was hard to believe, Muller said, that so little — just a pinch or two — could cause such misery. He had thought his head would split, and the pain in his legs had been almost beyond endurance. Dr. Levy returned him sympathetically to the night of March 27th. They had finished with the sausage around midnight, Muller remembered. The cook had departed by then, but his helpers were still at work. There had been five of them. He didn't know their names, but he had seen all or most of them again the next night, during the feast. Neither he nor Breit had given them any of the sausage before they left. But it was possible, of course, since the refrigerator in which he and Breit had stored the meat was not, like some, equipped with a lock . . . Dr. Levy thanked him, and moved rapidly to the door.

Dr. Levy spent the rest of the morning in the Bronx. After lunch, he hopped over to Queens. From there, he made his way to Brooklyn. It was past four by the time he got back to his office. He was hot and gritty from a dozen subway journeys, and his legs ached from pounding pavements and stairs and hospital corridors, but he had tracked down and had a revealing chat with each of Sauer's kitchen colleagues, and his heart was light. Three of them — William Ritter, Rudolf Nath, and Frederick Kreisler — were in hospitals. Ritter was at Fordham, Nath at Queens General, and Kreisler at the Coney Island Hospital, not far from his home in Brooklyn. The fourth member of the group, Henry Kuhn, was sick in bed at home. All were veterans of numerous reasonable but incorrect diagnoses, all were in more discomfort than danger, and all, it was obvious to Dr. Levy's unclouded eye, were suffering from trichinosis. Its source was equally obvious. They had prowled the icebox after the departure of Muller and Breit, come upon the sausage meat, and cheerfully helped themselves. They thought it was hamburger.

Before settling down at his desk to compose the final installment of his report, Dr. Levy looked in on Dr. Greenberg. He wanted, among other things, to relieve him of the agony of suspense. Dr. Greenberg gave him a chair, a cigarette, and an attentive ear. At the end of the travelogue, he groaned. "Didn't they even bother to cook it?" he asked.

"Yes, most of them did," Dr. Levy said. "They made it up into patties and fried them. Kuhn cooked his fairly well. A few minutes, at least. The others liked theirs rare. All except Sauer. He ate his raw."

"Oh," Dr. Greenberg said.

"Also," Dr. Levy added, "he ate two."

A Perverse, Ungrateful, Maleficent Malady

Gout has been making life miserable for a fairly large portion of the human race for at least four thousand years, and there is no good reason to believe that it will not continue to do so for a long time to come. Most medical men agree, in one of the profession's infrequent excursions toward unanimity, that gout is among the oldest of diseases. Some of them go even further; they believe that gout probably was the first serious physical disorder with which mankind was afflicted. In their opinion, it has been in existence ever since man became civilized enough to provide more than rudimentary satisfaction for his hunger and thirst. They regard gout as a corollary of progress and a symbol of a superior culture, like airsickness. Sufferers from gout occasionally find a scrap of comfort in this point of view. It is one of the few consolations they have.

The torments that the gouty are called upon to endure border on the intolerable. An attack of gout invariably is accompanied by prolonged and excruciating pain. "Screw up the vise as tightly as possible, and you have rheumatism," a gouty American physician named Morris Longstreth wrote in 1882. "Give it another turn, and that is gout." The peculiar agony of gout has also been acknowledged by the poets, one of whom — James Thomson, a minor-keyed Scotsman — wrote in a verse called "The Castle of Indolence":

> The sleepless gout here counts the crowing cocks,
> A wolf now gnaws him, now a serpent stings.

Thomas Sydenham, the greatest clinical physician of the seventeenth century and one of gout's most wretched victims, declared that while suffering from an attack he could not tolerate the weight of bedclothes on his throbbing foot "nor the shaking of the floor from a person's walking briskly thereon." Sydney Smith, the eighteenth-century clergyman and wit, observed, in a letter to a friend, "When I have the gout, I feel as if I was walking on my eyeballs." According to the testimony of victims who have experienced a wide variety of painful afflictions, the tortures of gout are exceeded only by those of migraine and *tic douloureux*, a disorder that affects one of the facial nerves. *Tic douloureux* can be cured by surgery, however, and sufferers from migraine can sometimes be relieved by more complicated methods. Gout is incurable. Its attacks are periodic, occurring, on the average, once or twice a year during the early stages of the affliction and more and more frequently as it takes a firmer hold. During an especially savage seizure, some victims have been known to long for death. But even this release is almost certain to be denied them, because the disease is rarely, if ever, fatal.

The gouty, unlike those stricken by other unshakable maladies, seldom achieve a state of Christian resignation. Gout tends to inflame their tempers. Some doctors have come to look upon extreme cantankerousness as a definite symptom of the disease. The spleen of the gouty is often directed against the disease itself. It is not uncommon for a gout sufferer to invest his malady with human characteristics. "Yes, yes," wrote Horace Walpole, who was one of the afflicted. "I know its ways and its Jesuitic evasions." Human beings have rarely been more bitterly abused than gout. Perhaps the most caustic of all attacks on the disease is contained in a treatise by George Herman Ellwanger, an otherwise uncelebrated upstate journalist, written in 1897. Gout, he stated, is "a perverse, ungrateful, maleficent malady, that delights upon the slightest pretext in assaulting vulnerable humanity at the most unseasonable hours and inconvenient times; an affliction that is especially prone to picket clubmen, physicians, poets, and heads of official departments; a stomachic metabasis that in some indeterminable, underhanded way is occasionally connected with the moderate use of certain wines and malt-liquors, though these be otherwise of an innocuous character . . . a stealthy, rancorous, irascible, mordacious disorder, masked under many forms, that continues to defy the science, skill, and pharmacopoeia of the medical profession. It is the charlock of maladies, that may thrive in every soil and will not be eradicated, — the wolf of diseases, with ensanguined fangs and encarmined jowl, who refuses to be baited even with asafoetida. . . . Its poison comes by heritage, its venom lurks in the wine-cup, its seeds are sown at the gatherings of good-cheer."

History records only one victim of gout whose disposition is said to have remained sunny during spells of the disease. That was John Milton, who, according to John Aubrey, an early biographer of the poet, "would be chearfull even in his gowtefitts, and sing." This is held by people who have gout to be one of the most suspect statements in English literature. Gout drives its victims into humiliating loneliness. Ordinarily, the sight of a man in nearly unendurable pain stirs his friends and loved ones to tender expressions of pity and murmurs of encouragement. Gout rarely evokes this humane response. People seem disinclined to pamper the gouty. Sydenham didn't say whether the members of his household refrained from stomping around in his bedroom, but the chances are that they did not. Practically everybody who is not afflicted with gout is comfortably, if perhaps incorrectly, persuaded that it has much in common with a hangover; that it is no more, in other words, than an extreme state of self-induced physiological dishevelment. William Cowper, the eighteenth-century British poet, shared this stern, ungenerous view. He referred to gout, which he happened not to suffer from, as "pangs arthritic that infest the toe of libertine excess." Dr. David Hosack, who practiced in New York during the early nineteenth century, felt much the same way. "Many have lost their gout with their fortunes," he noted crustily. He went on to say, with diminishing crispness, that by fortune he meant "its attendants, ease, indolence, luxury, and habits of intemperance, both in eating and drinking." Notions of this sort, which are widespread, cause some prosperous and sedentary gout sufferers to feel self-conscious when drinking anything but water or eating anything but the simplest food; the reactions of the less affluent, and of necessity more active, gouty, who are often teetotallers, and sometimes vegetarians as well, are usually less introverted. A further peculiarity of gout is that many people who do not suffer from it consider it droll. As Cowper implied, the disease generally settles in one of the toes. The left big toe is the one affected in most instances. This eccentricity of the affliction has a subtle appeal to a certain type of sense of humor. People have been known to laugh uproariously at the despairing groans of a patient with a throbbing toe.

Not all sufferers from gout are even fortunate enough to know what is the matter with them. In a large number of cases, this is not because they neglect to consult a doctor. Gout has always been a misunderstood disease, but not for several hundred years has it been as badly misunderstood as it is today. Dr. John H. Talbott, Professor of Medicine at the University of Buffalo, expressed the belief not long ago, in a monograph entitled "Gout," that there might be at least a third of a million gouty people in the United States. "It is safe to estimate," he added, "that only a portion of this number is diagnosed as gout and treated for same." Other experts agree with Dr. Talbott. "It is sometimes easier for the layman friend of the patient to suspect the presence of gout than the patient or his physician," Dr. Philip S. Hench, of the Mayo Clinic, lately reported. The Mayo Clinic, the University of Buffalo, the Massachusetts General Hospital, and the Presbyterian Hospital and Mount Sinai Hospital in New York City are the only institutions in the country where gout is currently the subject of serious investigation. Most contemporary physicians apparently regard it as old-fashioned to recognize this ancient disease when they see it. They prefer to think that they are tilting with more up-to-date and less stubborn ailments. In 1932, the *British Medical Journal* announced joyfully that "gout is an almost extinct disease." These glad, if somewhat impulsive, tidings were accepted with relief and alacrity in this country as well as in England by practically all members of the profession except the gout specialists. Several of the latter felt impelled to protest. "Fashions in therapy may have some justification, fashions in diagnosis have none," Dr. W. W.

Herrick and Dr. T. Lloyd Tyson, members of the faculty of the Columbia University College of Physicians and Surgeons, who had encountered a great deal of gout, complained in the *American Journal of the Medical Sciences.* "Strangely enough, acute gout, one of the oldest maladies known to medicine, seems almost to have become one of the forgotten diseases. Here is a definite clinical entity of which there is ample description and record and which in its ordinary manifestations is easy of recognition; and yet it seems to have become the fashion persistently to ignore it in the differential diagnosis of the arthritides. Is this not another example of the closing of the mind to the obvious — a fault that so seriously besets all medical diagnosis?"

Some doctors appear to have managed to close their minds to the obvious almost indefinitely. Dr. Abraham Cohen, Chief of the Arthritis Clinic at the Philadelphia General Hospital, has reported that during a five-year study he came across forty cases of well-advanced gout, six of which, though under medical observation, had run on for more than twenty years without being properly diagnosed. The most fashionable error in diagnosis at the moment is to confuse gout with one or another of the more elaborate forms of arthritis, a disease to which it is, as a matter of fact, related. Some doctors who are persuaded that gout is an anachronism merely diagnose it as a sprain or an infection and cause their patients unnecessary torment by applying the customary methods of treating such ailments. Occasionally these cases of mistaken identity approach the spectacular. One instance of this sort recently came to the attention of Drs. Herrick and Tyson. "Mr. W. A. M., aged fifty-five," they subsequently wrote, "complained of attacks . . . in the ankles, knees, and great toes, at intervals, for twelve years. With each, a newly infected tooth had been found and removed." Mr. W. A. M., it turned out, was suffering from gout, which has nothing to do with the condition of the teeth. A year or two ago, repeated encounters with clumsy diagnoses prompted three Boston physicians — Dr. Joseph P. McCracken, Dr. Philip S. Owen, and Dr. Joseph H. Pratt — to offer their fellow-subscribers to the A. M. A. *Journal* a handy pointer on the recognition of gout. "Acute inflammation of the first metatarsophalangeal joint almost always means gout and should be so treated," they wrote. (The first metatarsophalangeal joint is in the big toe.) "Unless the disease is recognized," they added, with perhaps unconscious tartness, "adequate treatment is impossible."

Although gout cannot be cured, the severity of its periodic attacks can be lessened and their duration greatly shortened by treatment involving the use of a drug called colchicum, which is obtained from meadow saffron, or *Colchicum autumnale*. Colchicum was discovered by the ancient Greeks and named by them for Colchis, the country in Asia Minor where Medea is supposed to have practiced her black arts and where meadow saffron was first found. The drug is a powerful diuretic and cathartic, and a vicious poison. It is also a specific for gout, but it has no known effect on any other disease. In this, it differs from practically all other drugs. Its potency is staggering. Gram for gram colchicum is seven hundred times more potent than aspirin. An untreated attack of gout often lasts as long as two weeks. Colchicum usually ends an attack within forty-eight hours. Just how colchicum goes about doing this, doctors do not know. One reason they do not is that the cause of gout is not known.

The dossier on gout is, nevertheless, a fairly thick one.

Gout is believed to be primarily, if not exclusively, a familial ailment. It is also believed to be essentially a metabolic disease. The human body normally contains a small amount of uric acid, a chemical substance that is produced during the digestion of certain foods and alcoholic beverages. An abnormal amount of uric acid in the body is a symptom of gout. Most physicians who are familiar with gout, however, are certain that uric acid is no more the basic cause of gout than sugar is the basic cause of diabetes. On the other hand, such experts say, if a person comes from a gouty family, and is therefore presumably susceptible to gout, an increase in the amount of uric acid in his system will probably precipitate an attack, just as will the introduction of sugar into the blood stream of a diabetic. Uric acid is non-toxic. In the course of treating other diseases, large quantities of it have been injected into the veins of people with no known gouty forbears and no sign of the disease has developed. Uric acid is, to be sure, the direct cause of the physical crippling that sometimes develops in cases of advanced gout, for it has a way of forming crystalline deposits in the joints of the arms and legs, but since these deposits do not appear until the patient has been a sufferer for many years, the pain by which all gouty people are tormented cannot very well be attributed to them. Nobody knows what causes the pain of gout.

The hereditary nature of gout may have been suspected by Mother Goose (whose works, as it happens, mention no other disease) when she wrote:

> Lazy Tom with jacket blue,
> Stole his father's gouty shoe.
> The worst of harm that Dad can wish him,
> Is his gouty shoe may fit him.

Charles Dickens sensed the hereditary nature of gout, too. In "Bleak House," he says of Sir Leicester Dedlock that he "yields up his family legs to the family disorder, as if he held his name and fortune on that feudal tenure." Sir Leicester's acceptance of his unhappy heritage was an unusually philosophical one. A more human reaction was recorded by James Russell Lowell. "I call my gout the unearned increment from my good grandfather's Madeira," he wrote, "and think how excellent it must have been, and sip it cool from the bin of fancy, and wish he had left me the cause instead of the effect." There is no convincing evidence that gout ever afflicts those who have no inherited predisposition to it. (This does not, unfortunately, explain how the disease got started in the first place.) Gout, like baldness, is one of the misfortunes of masculinity and advancing age. Women hardly ever get it, and only rarely does a man under forty come down with it. Gout also has an unmistakable seasonal incidence. Its victims are most often taken in the early months of the year and in the autumn. Another of the cheerless idiosyncrasies of the disease is that its attacks generally begin an hour or two after midnight. "The regular gout," Sydenham noted in his relentlessly autobiographical "A Treatise of the Gout," "seizes in the following manner: It comes on a sudden towards the close of January, or the beginning of February, giving scarce any sign of its approach. . . . The day preceding the fit the appetite is sharp, but preternatural. The patient goes to bed, and sleeps quietly, till about two in the morning, when he is awakened by a pain, which usually seizes the great toe."

The traditional treatment of gout requires that all foods and beverages highly conducive to the formation of uric acid be firmly avoided. This calls for a heartless regimen.

The diet excludes almost every item of food and drink that makes life worth living — meat, game, fowl, fish, gravy, butter, cheese, nuts, mince pie, many vegetables, most soups, rum, brandy, wine, beer, whiskey, gin, and even Wheaties. Some doctors proscribe coffee and tea as well. The gouty are advised to dine as best they can on such plain fare as eggs, grits, dandelion greens, white bread, and potatoes. They may also, if they wish, nibble caviar and zwieback. "If it be objected that a total abstinence from wine and other fermented liquors would render life in a manner insupportable," Sydenham noted wistfully, "I answer, it must be considered." A century or so ago, doctors seemed concerned more with keeping their gouty patients sober than with keeping them undernourished. Sir Alfred Garrod, a prominent nineteenth-century specialist, adopted an almost Volsteadian implacability in this regard. "The use of fermented liquors is the most powerful of all the predisposing causes of gout," he wrote, "nay, so powerful, that it may be a question whether gout would ever have been known to mankind had such beverages not been indulged in." Contemporary authorities are beginning to take a somewhat more tolerant view toward drink, and they are far from sure that diet makes much difference. They have not, however, wholly rejected the idea that some relationship exists between gout and gracious living. In the encouragement of gout-sufferers who chafe at austerity, the furthest that Dr. Talbott, for one, will go is to suggest that there are several agents more likely than self-indulgence to bring on an attack. "These include," he recently noted, "drugs, trauma, acute infections, and surgical operations."

The first known treatment of gout consisted of burning flax near the affected joint, presumably to smoke out the trouble. Hippocrates advocated this innocent therapy in the third century B.C. He is the first physician of record to have recognized gout as a generic disease, and certain of his clinical observations on its seasonal aspects, its striking affinity for males, and its seeming connection with eating and drinking are still more or less valid. He called the disease *podagra,* a Greek word which means a snare for the feet. The term "gout" did not appear until the thirteenth century. It is derived from the Latin *gutta,* meaning "drop," and was hit upon because of a belief, prevalent at the time, that the pain of gout was caused by a poison that entered the afflicted joint drop by drop. In one of the few surviving manuscripts of that period, "The Early South English Legendary, or Lives of the Saints," there is a reference to the affliction: "There cam a goute In is kneo, of Anguische gret . . . So longue, that is kneo to swal."

Hippocrates' strategy of fighting gout with flax smoke seems to have remained in vogue for nearly eight hundred years. Then, about 500 A.D., a Mesopotamian physician named Aëtius, a man, it would seem, of almost unlimited whimsicality, began recommending a month-by-month program for sufferers from the disease who wished to avoid further attacks. "In January," he advised: "take a glass of pure wine every morning; February: eat no beets; March: mix sweets with eatables and drinkables; April: refrain from horse radish; May: eat no polypus fishes; June: take cold water every morning; July: abstain from venery; August: eat no mallows; September: drink only milk; October: garlic must be eaten; November: bathing is prohibited; December: eat freely of cabbage." How effective the Aëtius treatment proved to be is not known, but it was generally supplanted half a century later by a formula that a Greek doctor, Alexander of Tralles, worked out. This called for a mixture of caraway seeds, anise, rhubarb, wolf's milk, vinegar, honey, dill, pepper, ginger, aloes, and — pretty much by chance — colchicum. As a result of the colchicum, Alexander got some sensationally successful results, but unfortunately he had included the drug simply as a purge and before long substituted a less violent one.

During the Middle Ages, when the science of medicine reached a state of confusion unequalled even in the more backward cultures along the upper Amazon, many doctors managed to outdo Aëtius in the capriciousness of their remedies. A seventeenth-century Prussian doctor named Daniel Sennert, who was one of the less gifted colleagues of William Harvey, the discoverer of the fact that blood circulates, took to treating gout by applying to the afflicted joint a poultice composed of marsh-mallow leaves, cabbage, barley, and frog sperm. At about the same time, John Loselius, a German physician who seems to have been a naturalist at heart, offered his patients more excitement for their money. "Shave with a razor the hair off both legs," he recommended, "and at the same time cut the nails of hands and feet. This should be in the spring when the sap is flowing, and the day before new moon. Make a hole right into the heartwood of a poplar or oak tree and insert the hair and nails. Stop it tight with a plug made of a branch of the tree, and the transplantation is perfect. Cut off close to the tree that part of the plug that sticks out, and the next day plaster the place well with cow dung. If the patient does not in the next three months feel the *malum* again," he added, sidestepping quickly, "he can credit it to the tree." Many English and French physicians in the early eighteenth century believed that gout could be cured by a touch of the hand of George I or Louis XIV. The inability of the latter, who was a lifelong sufferer from gout, to cure himself undoubtedly led to some awkward moments at medical get-togethers. In 1735, Sir Richard Blackmore, a pioneer Coué, announced that gout was all in the mind. "Fright can cause and cure an attack," he said, and turned his attention to something else. It was not until 1763 that colchicum's effectiveness in relieving gout sufferers was detected. Baron von Stoerck, of Vienna, is generally credited with this discovery. The drug was introduced to this country by Benjamin Franklin, who had a terrible time with gout and got wind of the colchicum treatment during his stay in France.

Gout seems always to have had a special fondness for men of consequence. Alexander the Great and Kubla Khan had it. So did Ben Jonson, Talleyrand, Martin Luther, John Wesley, Henry Fielding, Edward Gibbon, Thomas Gray, Stendhal, Sir Isaac Newton, Samuel Johnson, the Pitts (father and son), William Congreve, Francis Bacon, William Harvey, Lord Tennyson, Walter Savage Landor, Charles Darwin, General Winfield Scott, Guy de Maupassant, and John Barrymore. The idea that gout has a habit of striking in the upper brackets of accomplishment appealed strongly to Sydenham. "But indeed in this manner have lived, and in this manner have finally died, majestic Kings, Rulers, Generals, Philosophers, and Admirals, and many others of like rank," he wrote in his masterwork. "Briefly, I should assert that this gout (and you can hardly affirm as much of any other malady) slays more of the Rich than the Poor, and rather the Wise than the Fool."

Many reflective, and in some cases gouty, physicians have since sided with Sydenham on this point. In support of the thesis, Dr. William Cullen, a nineteenth-century Londoner, was impressed to discover that gout very frequently attacked "men of large heads," and a contemporary fellow-countryman, Dr. Chalmers Watson, satisfied himself that gout is "peculiarly incidental to men of cultivated mind and intellectual distinction." No one, though, has pursued the thought further or with more spirit than Dr. Havelock Ellis. "There is . . . a pathological condition which occurs so often, in such extreme forms, in men of such preëminent intellectual ability, that it is impossible not to regard it as having a real association with such ability," he wrote in "A Study of British Genius." "I refer to gout." Ellis, an objective, or non-gouty, observer, based his conclusions on his contention that of the people "most commonly mentioned by national biographers," more suffered from gout than from any other disease. "This association of ability and gout," he continued, "cannot be a fortuitous coincidence. The genius of the gouty group is emphatically masculine, profoundly original; these men show a massive and patient energy. . . . Not only is the gouty poison itself probably an irritant and stimulant to the nervous system, but even its fluctuations may be mentally beneficial. When it is in the victim's blood, his brain becomes abnormally overclouded, if not intoxicated; when it is in his joints, his mind becomes abnormally clear and vigorous." Gathering speed and confidence, Ellis went on in this vein at some length, and only when he reached his peroration did he brake himself slightly. "It must not, in any case, be supposed that in thus suggesting a real connection between gout and genius it is thereby assumed that the latter is in any sense a product of the former," he warned. "It may well be, however, that, given a highly endowed and robust organism, the gouty poison acts as a real stimulus to intellectual ability, and a real aid in intellectual achievement."

A while ago, someone asked Dr. Alexander B. Gutman, a highly endowed and robust organism, who is directing the research work on gout at Mount Sinai Hospital, if he thought that an occasional gouty spasm might help sharpen his wits and thus speed the successful completion of his task. Dr. Gutman, who does not happen to have gout, winced and said he doubted it. "We know what the main substances that the brain uses for food are," he said, "and uric acid isn't one of them. Also, we have no evidence at all that a pain in the toe stimulates the mind."

A Game of Wild Indians

DURING the second week in August, 1946, an elderly man, a middle-aged woman, and a boy of ten dragged themselves, singly and painfully, into the Presbyterian Hospital, in the Washington Heights section of Manhattan, where their trouble was unhesitatingly identified as typhoid fever. This diagnosis was soon confirmed by laboratory analysis, and on Thursday morning, August 15th, a report of the outbreak was dutifully telephoned to the Department of Health. It was received and recorded there, in accordance with the routine in all alarms of an epidemiological nature, by a clerk in the Bureau of Preventable Diseases named Beatrice Gamso. Miss Gamso is a low-strung woman and she has spent some thirty callousing years in the Health Department, but the news gave her a turn. She sat for an instant with her eyes on her notes. Then, steadying herself with a practiced hand, she swung around to her typewriter and set briskly about dispatching copies of the report to all administrative officers of the Department. Within an hour, a reliable investigator from the Bureau was on his way to Washington Heights. He was presently followed by one of his colleagues, a Department public-health nurse, several agents from the Bureau of Food and Drugs, and an inspector from the Bureau of Sanitary Engineering.

Typhoid fever was among the last of the massive pestilential fevers to yield to the probings of medical science, but its capitulation has been complete. It is wholly transparent now. Its clinical manifestations (a distinctive rash and a tender spleen, a fiery fever and a languid pulse, and nausea, diarrhea, and nosebleed), its cause (a bacillus known as *Eberthella typhosa*), and its means of transmission have all been clearly established. Typhoid is invariably conveyed by food or drink contaminated with the excreta of its victims. Ordinarily, it is spread by someone who is ignorant, at least momentarily, of his morbid condition. One reason for such unawareness is that for the first several days typhoid fever tends to be disarmingly mild and indistinguishable from the countless fleeting malaises that dog the human race. Another is that nearly five per cent of the cases become typhoid carriers, continuing indefinitely to harbor a lively colony of typhoid bacilli in their systems. The existence of typhoid carriers was discovered by a group of German hygienists in 1907. Typhoid Mary Mallon, a housemaid and cook who was the stubborn cause of a total of fifty-three cases in and around New York City a generation ago, is, of course, the most celebrated of these hapless menaces. About seventy per cent, by some unexplained physiological fortuity, are women. The names of three hundred and eighty local carriers are currently on active file in the Bureau of Preventable Diseases. They are called on regularly by public-health nurses and are permanently enjoined from any employment that involves the handling of food. More than a third of all the cases that occur here are traced to local carriers but, because of the vigilance of the Health Department, rarely to recorded carriers; new ones keep turning up. Most of the rest of the cases are of unknown or out-of-town origin. A few are attributable to the products of polluted waters (clams and oysters and various greens).

The surveillance of carriers is one of several innovations that in little more than a generation have forced typhoid fever into an abrupt tractability throughout most of the Western world. The others include certain refinements in diagnostic technique, the institution of public-health measures requiring the chlorination of city-supplied water and proscribing the sale of unpasteurized milk, and the development of an immunizing vaccine. Since late in the nineteenth century, the local incidence of typhoid fever has dropped from five or six thousand cases a year to fewer than fifty, and it is very possible that it may soon be as rare as smallpox. Banishment has not, however, materially impaired the vigor of *Eberthella typhosa*. Typhoid fever is still a cruel and withering affliction. It is always rambunctious, generally prolonged, and often fatal. It is also one of the most explosive of communicable diseases. The month in which it is most volcanic is August.

The investigator who led the sprint to Washington Heights that August morning in 1946 was Dr. Harold T. Fuerst, an epidemiologist, and he and Dr. Ottavio J. Pellitteri, another epidemiologist, handled most of the medical inquiry. One afternoon, when I was down at the Bureau, they told me about the case. Miss Gamso sat at a desk nearby, and I noticed after a moment that she was following the conversation with rapt attention. Her interest, it turned out, was entirely understandable. Typhoid-fever investigations are frequently tedious, but they are seldom protracted. It is not unusual for a team of experienced operatives to descry the source of an outbreak in a couple of days. Some cases have been riddled in an afternoon. The root of the trouble on Washington Heights eluded detection for almost two weeks, and it is probable that but for Miss Gamso it would never have been detected at all.

"I got to Presbyterian around eleven," Dr. Fuerst told me. "I found a staff man I knew, and he led me up to the patients. It was typhoid, all right. Not that I'd doubted it, but it's routine to take a look. And they were in bad shape — too miserable to talk. One — the woman — was barely conscious. I decided to let the questioning go for the time being. At least until I'd seen their histories. A clerk in the office of the medical superintendent dug them out for me. Pretty skimpy — name, age, sex, occupation, and address, and a few clinical notations. About all I got at a glance was that they weren't members of the same family. I'd hoped, naturally, that they would be. That would have nicely limited the scope of the investigation. Then I noticed something interesting. They weren't a family, but they had a little more in common than just typhoid. For one thing, they were by way of being neighbors. One of them lived at 502 West 180th Street, another at 501 West 178th Street, and the third at 285 Audubon Avenue, just around the corner from where it runs through the five-hundred block of West 179th Street. Another thing was their surnames. They were different, but they weren't dissimilar. All three were of Armenian origin. Well, Washington Heights has an Armenian colony — very small and very clannish. I began to feel pretty good. I didn't doubt for a minute that the three of them knew each other. Quite possibly they were friends. If so, it was reasonable to suppose that they might recently have shared a meal. It wasn't very likely, of course, that they had been the only ones to share it. Ten-year-old boys don't usually go out to meals without their parents. Maybe there had been a dozen in on it. It could even have been some sort of national feast. Or a church picnic. Picnic food is an ideal breeding ground for the typhoid organism. It can't stand cooking, but it thrives in raw stuff — ice cream and mayonnaise and so on. And if a carrier had happened to have a hand in the arrangements . . . I decided we'd do well to check and see if there was an Armenian carrier on our list."

"We found one, all right," Dr. Pellitteri said. "A widow named Christos — she died a year or two ago — who lived on West 178th Street."

"To be sure, we had only three cases," Dr. Fuerst went on. "But I didn't let that bother me. I've never known an outbreak of typhoid in which everybody who was exposed got sick. There are always a certain number who escape. They either don't eat whatever it is that's contaminated or they have a natural or an acquired immunity. Moreover, the incubation period in typhoid — the time it takes for the bug to catch hold — varies with the individual. Ten days is about the average, but it can run anywhere from three to thirty. In other words, maybe we had seen only the vanguard. There might be more to come. So in the absence of anything better, the Armenian link looked pretty good. I called the Bureau and told Bill Birnkrant — he was acting director at the time — what I thought, and he seemed to think the same. He said he'd start somebody checking. I went back upstairs for another try at the patients."

"That's when the rest of us began to come into the picture," Dr. Pellitteri said. "My job was the recent social life of the Armenian colony. Ida Matthews, a public-health nurse, took the carrier angle. Neither of us had much luck. The file listed twelve carriers in Washington Heights. As I remember, the only Armenian was Mrs. Christos. At any rate, the nurse picked her first. I remember running into Miss Matthews somewhere on Audubon toward the end of that first afternoon. She told me what progress she had made. None. Mrs. Christos was old and sick, and hadn't been out of her apartment for a month. Miss Matthews said there was no reason to doubt the woman's word, as she had a good reputation at the Department — very coöperative, obeyed all the rules. Miss Matthews was feeling pretty gloomy. She'd had high hopes. Well, I knew how she felt. I'd hit nothing but dead ends myself. Our patients didn't seem to be friends. Apparently, they just knew each other. The priest at the Gregorian church in the neighborhood — Holy Cross Armenian Apostolic, on West 187th Street — knew of no recent feasts or festivals. He hadn't heard of any unusual amount of illness in the parish, either. No mysterious chills and fevers. And the Armenian doctors in the neighborhood said the same. They had seen nothing that resembled typhoid except the cases we already had. Before I gave up for the day, I even got in touch with an Armenian girl who used to work at the Department. The only thing I could think of at the moment was a check of the Armenian restaurants. When I mentioned that, she burst out laughing. It seems Armenians don't frequent Armenian restaurants. They prefer home cooking."

"I got Pellitteri's report the next morning," Dr. Fuerst said. "And Miss Matthews'." I was back at the hospital, and when I called Birnkrant, he gave me the gist of them. I can't say I was greatly surprised. To tell the truth, I was relieved. The Armenian picnic I'd hypothesized the day before would have created a real mess. Because the hospital had reported two new cases. Two women. They lived at 500 West 178th Street and 611 West 180th Street, but they weren't Armenians. One was Italian. The other was plain American. So we were right back where we started. Only, now we had five cases instead of three, and nothing to tie them together but the fact that they all lived in the same neighborhood. And had the same brand of typhoid. There are around a dozen different strains, you know, which sometimes complicates matters. About the only thing Birnkrant and I could be sure of was that the feast theory — any kind of common gathering — was out. I'd had a word with the new patients. They had never even heard of each other. So the link had to be indirect. That gave us a number of possibilities. The source of infection could be water — either drinking water or a swimming pool. Or it could be commercial ice. Or milk. Or food. Drinking water was a job for Sanitary Engineering. The others, at the moment, were up to us — meaning Pellitteri and me. They were all four conceivable. Even ice. You can find a precedent for anything and everything in the literature on typhoid. But just one was probable. That was food. Some food that is sold already prepared — like potato salad or frozen custard — or one that is usually eaten raw. All we had to do was find out what it was, and where they got it, and how it got that way. Birnkrant and I figured out the area involved. It came to roughly four square blocks. I don't know if you know that part of Washington Heights. It's no prairie. Every building is a big apartment house, and the ground floors of most are stores. At least a fourth have something to do with food."

"I was in the office when Fuerst called," Dr. Pellitteri said. "Before he hung up, I got on the phone and we made the necessary arrangements about questioning the patients and their families — who was to see who. Then I took off. I wasn't too pessimistic. The odds were against a quick answer, but you never know. It was just possible that they all bought from the same store. Well, as it happened, they did. In a way. The trouble was it wasn't one store. It was practically all of them. Fuerst had the same experience. We ended up at the office that evening with a list as long as my arm — half a dozen fruit-and-vegetable stands, four or five groceries, a market that sold clams, and an assortment of ice-cream parlors and confectioneries and delicatessens. Moreover, we couldn't even be sure the list included the right store. Most people have very strange memories. They forget and they imagine. You've got to assume that most of the information they give you may be either incomplete or inaccurate, or both. But there *was* a right store — we knew that. Sanitary Engineering had eliminated drinking water, and we had been able to rule out swimming and milk and ice. Only one of the group ever went swimming, all but one family had electric refrigerators, and none of them had drunk unpasteurized milk. It had to be contaminated food from a store. That much was certain."

"It was also certain that we had to have some help," Dr. Fuerst said. "Pellitteri and I could have handled a couple of stores. Or even, at a pinch, three or four. But a dozen or more — it would take us weeks. Let me give you an idea what an investigation like that involves. You don't just walk in the store and gaze around. You more or less take it apart. Every item of food that could conceivably cause trouble is examined, the physical setup is inspected for possible violations of the Sanitary Code, and all employees and their families are interviewed and specimens taken for laboratory analysis. So we needed help, and, of course, we got it. Birnkrant had a conference with the Commissioner the next morning and they talked it over, and the result was an engineer and another nurse and a fine big team from Food and Drugs. Very gratifying."

"And Miss Matthews," Dr. Pellitteri said. "We had her back again. She had finally finished with her carriers. They were all like the first. None had violated any of the rules."

"As expected," Dr. Fuerst said. "The average carrier is pretty coöperative. Well, that was Saturday. By Monday, we had made a certain amount of progress. We hadn't found anything yet, but the field was narrowing down. And all of a sudden we got a little nibble. It came from a confectionery called Pop's, on 178th Street, around noon. Pop's had been well up on our list. They sold ice cream made on the premises, and the place was a neighborhood favorite. Which meant it got a very thorough going over. But we were about ready to cross it off — everything was in good shape, including the help — when it developed that the place had just changed hands. Pop had sold out a week before, and he and his wife, who'd helped him run it, were on the way to California. Needless to say, Pop's went back on the list, and at the top. Also, somebody did some quick checking. Pop and his wife were driving, and their plan was to spend a few days with friends in Indianapolis. That gave us a chance. We called Birnkrant and he called Indianapolis — the State Health Department. They were extremely interested. Naturally. They said they'd let us know."

Dr. Fuerst lighted a cigarette. "Then we got a jolt," he said. "Several, in fact. The first was a call from the hospital. Four new cases. That brought the total up to nine. But it didn't stay there long. Tuesday night, it went to ten. I don't mind saying that set us back on our heels. Ten cases of typhoid fever in less than a week in one little corner of the city is almost unheard of in this day and age. The average annual incidence for the whole of Washington Heights is hardly half a case. That wasn't the worst of it, though. The real blow was that tenth case. I'll call him Jones. Jones didn't fit in. The four Monday cases, like the three Armenians and the Italian and the American, all lived in that one four-block area. Jones didn't. He lived on 176th Street, but way over west, almost on Riverside Drive. An entirely different neighborhood. I had a word with Jones the first thing Wednesday morning. I remember he worked for the post office. That's about all I learned. He hardly knew where he was. When I left the hospital, I called on his wife. She wasn't much help, either. She did all the family marketing, she told me, and she did it all within a block or two of home. That was that. She was very definite. On the other hand, there was Mr. Jones. He had typhoid, which doesn't just happen, and it was the same strain as all the rest. So either it was a very strange coincidence or she was too upset to think. My preference, until proved otherwise, was the latter. I found a phone, and called Birnkrant and gave him the latest news. He had some news for me. Indianapolis had called. They had located Pop and his wife and made the usual tests. The results were negative."

"I don't know which was the most discouraging," Dr. Pellitteri said. "Jones, I guess. He meant more work — a whole new string of stores to check. Pop had been ninety per cent hope. He merely aroused suspicion. He ran a popular place, he sold homemade ice cream, and when the epidemic broke, he pulled out. Or so it appeared from where we stood. It hurt to lose him. Unlikely or not, he had been a possibility — the first specific lead of any kind that we had been able to find in a week of mighty hard work. During the next few days, it began to look more and more like the last. Until Friday evening. Friday evening we got a very excited call from the laboratory. It was about a batch of specimens we had submitted that morning for analysis. One of them was positive for *E. typhosa.* The man's name doesn't matter. It didn't even then. What did matter was his occupation. He was the proprietor of a little frozen-custard shop — now extinct — that I'll call the Jupiter. The location was interesting, too. It was a trifle outside our area, but still accessible, and a nice, easy walk from the Joneses'. Food and Drugs put an embargo on the Jupiter that night. The next morning, we began to take it apart."

"I missed that," Dr. Fuerst said. "I spent Saturday at the hospital. It was quite a day. We averaged a case an hour. I'm not exaggerating. When I finally left, the count was nine. Nine brand-new cases. A couple of hours later, one more turned up. That made twenty, all told. Fortunately, that was the end. Twenty was the grand total. But, of course, we didn't know that then. There was no reason to believe they wouldn't just keep coming."

"The rest of us had the same kind of day," Dr. Pellitteri said. "Very disagreeable. There was the owner of the Jupiter — poor devil. You can imagine the state he was in. All of a sudden, he was out of business and a public menace. He didn't even know what a typhoid carrier was. He had to be calmed down and instructed. That was the beginning. It got worse. First of all, the Jupiter was as clean as a whistle. We closed it up — had to, under the circumstances — and embargoed the stock, but we didn't find anything. That was peculiar. I can't explain it even now. He was either just naturally careful or lucky. While that was going on, we went back to the patients and questioned them again. Did they know the Jupiter? Were they customers? Did they ever buy anything there? We got one yes. The rest said no. Emphatically. If there had been a few more yeses — even three or four — we might have wondered. But they couldn't all be mistaken. So the Jupiter lead began to look pretty wobbly. Then the laboratory finished it off. They had a type report on the Jupiter organism. It wasn't the *E. typhosa* we were looking for. It was one of the other strains. That may have been some consolation to Mr. Jupiter. At least, he didn't have an epidemic on his conscience. But it left us uncomfortably close to the end of our rope. We had only a handful of stores still to check. If we didn't find the answer there, we were stumped. We didn't. We crossed off the last possibility on Tuesday morning, August 27th. It was Number Eighty. We'd examined eighty stores and something like a thousand people, and all we had to show for it was a new carrier."

"Well, that was something," Dr. Fuerst said. "Even if it was beside the point. But we also had another consolation. None of the patients had died. None was going to. They were all making excellent progress."

"That's true enough," Dr. Pellitteri said. "But we couldn't claim much credit for that." He paused, and shifted around in his chair. "About all we can take any credit for is Miss Gamso, here," He smiled. "Miss Gamso saved the day. She got inspired."

Miss Gamso gave me a placid look. "I don't know about inspired," she said. "It was more like annoyed. I heard them talking — Dr. Birnkrant, and these two, and all the rest of them — and I read the reports, and the days went by and they didn't seem to be getting anywhere. That's unusual. So it was irritating. It's hard to explain, but I got to thinking about that carrier Mrs. Christos. There were two things about her. She lived with a son-in-law who was a known food handler. He was a baker by trade. Also, where she lived was right in the middle of everything — 519 West 178th Street. That's just off Audubon. And Audubon is the street where practically all our cases did most of their shopping. Well, there was one store in particular — a fruit-and-vegetable market called Tony's — on almost everybody's list. The address was 261 Audubon Avenue. Then I really got a brainstorm. It was right after lunch on Tuesday, August 27th. I picked up the telephone and called the bureau that registers house numbers at the Borough President's office, and I asked them one question. Did 519 West 178th Street and 261 Audubon Avenue happen by any chance to be the same building? They asked me why I wanted to know. I wasn't talking, though. I just said was it, in a nice way, and the man finally said he'd see. When he came back, I was right. They were one and the same. I was so excited I thought I'd burst. Dr. Pellitteri was sitting right where he is now. He was the first person I saw, so I marched straight over and told him. He kind of stared at me. He had the funniest expression." Miss Ganso smiled a gentle smile. "I think he thought I'd gone crazy."

"I wouldn't say that," Dr. Pellitteri said. "I'll admit, however, that I didn't quite see the connection. We'd been all over Tony's — it was almost our first stop — and there was no earthly reason to question Miss Matthews' report on Mrs. Christos. The fact that they occupied the same building was news to me. To all of us, as I recall. But what if they did? Miss Gamso thought it was significant or suspicious or something. The point escaped me. When she mentioned the son-in-law, though, I began to get a little more interested. We knew him, of course — anybody who lives with a carrier is a potential cause of trouble — and checked on him regularly. But it was just possible that since our last checkup he had become infected. That happens. And although we hadn't found him working in any of the stores, he could have come and gone a couple of weeks before we started our investigation. At any rate, it was worth looking into. Almost anything was, by then. I went up that afternoon. I walked past Tony's on the way to 519. There wasn't any doubt about their being in the same building. Tony's is gone now, like Mrs. Christos, but the way it was then, his front door was about three steps from the corner, and around the corner about three more steps was the entrance to the apartments above. The Christos flat was on the fifth floor — Apartment 53. Mrs. Christos and her son-in-law were both at home. They let me in and that's about all. I can't say they were either one delighted to see me. Or very helpful. She couldn't add anything to what she had already told Miss Matthews. The son-in-law hardly opened his mouth. His last regular job, he said, had been in January, in a cafeteria over in Astoria. Since then, he'd done nothing but odd jobs. He wouldn't say what, when, or where. I couldn't completely blame him. He was afraid that if we got to questioning any of his former employers, they'd never take him on again. When I saw how it was, I arranged for a specimen and, for the moment, let it go at that. There was no point in getting rough until we knew for sure. I told him to sit tight. If he was positive, I'd be back in a hurry. I got the report the next day. He wasn't. He was as harmless as I am. But by then it didn't matter. By that time, it was all over. To tell the truth, I had the answer before I ever left the building."

Dr. Pellitteri shook his head. "I walked right into it," he said. "It was mostly pure luck. What happened was this. On the way out, I ran into the superintendent — an elderly woman. I was feeling two ways about the son-in-law — half sympathetic and half suspicious. It occurred to me that the superintendent might have some idea where he'd been working the past few weeks. So I stopped and asked. She was a sour old girl. She didn't know and didn't care. She had her own troubles. They were the tenants, mainly. She backed me into a corner and proceeded to unload. The children were the worst, she said — especially the boys. Always thinking up some new devilment. For example, she said, just a few weeks ago, toward the end of July, there was a gang of them up on the roof playing wild Indians. Before she could chase them off, they'd stuffed some sticks down one of the plumbing vent pipes. The result was a stoppage. The soil pipe serving one whole tier of apartments blocked and sprang a leak, and the bathroom of the bottom apartment was a nice mess. I hadn't been paying much attention until then. But at that point — Well, to put it mildly, I was fascinated. Also, I began to ask some questions. I wanted to know just what bathroom had flooded. The answer was Apartment 23. What were the other apartments in that tier? They were 33, 43, and 53. What was underneath Apartment 23? A store — Tony's Market, on the corner. Then I asked for a telephone. Birnkrant's reaction was about what you'd expect. Pretty soon, a team from Sanitary Engineering arrived. They supplied the details and the proof. Tony stored his fruits and vegetables in a big wooden walk-in refrigerator at the rear of his store. When Sanitary Engineering pulled off the top, they found the soil pipe straight overhead. The leak had been repaired almost a month before, but the sawdust insulation in the refrigerator roof was still damp from the waste that had soaked through. It wasn't Tony's fault. He hadn't known. It wasn't anybody's fault. It was just one of those things. So that was that."

"Not entirely," Dr. Fuerst said. "There was still Jones to account for. It wasn't necessary. The thing was settled. But I was curious. I had a talk with him the next day. We talked and talked. And in the end, he remembered. He was a night walker. Every evening after dinner, he went out for a walk. He walked all over Washington Heights, and usually, somewhere along the line, he stopped and bought something to eat. It was generally a piece of fruit. As I say, he finally remembered. One night, near the end of July, he was walking down Audubon and he came to a fruit stand and he bought an apple. On the way home, he ate it."

The Alerting of Mr. Pomerantz

A VIOLENT, body-racking, infectious fever called rickettsialpox is the newest of known diseases. Its onset is abrupt, it is as prostrating as a kick in the stomach, and its course is a trying one, but it is not fatal. Although medical authorities are of the uneasy opinion that thousands of new diseases would afflict mankind if all the microörganisms potentially capable of causing illness were to become sufficiently virulent to break down the body's resistance to them, the outbreak of just one such disease is happily an unusual occurrence. The first known case of rickettsialpox in medical history turned up in the winter of 1946, in New York City. Cases of it have since been reported elsewhere in the country. No other disease has ever made its initial appearance here. It is, in fact, practically unheard of for one to originate in any metropolis. Nobody knows why.

Almost everything about rickettsialpox is peculiar. It is among the few identified ailments that bear scientifically illuminating names. A disease usually is named for its discoverer (Bright's disease), for the geographical area in which it was first observed (Asiatic cholera), or for its predominant symptom (whooping cough). Sometimes a disease is named for its cause or, as often as not, for what was once erroneously *thought* to be its cause (malaria, which is not caused by bad air, and the common cold, which is not caused by low temperatures). Rickettsialpox, as a name, not only gives a good idea of one of the disease's most notable manifestations, a spotty rash, but indicates its cause, a microörganism of the genus *Rickettsia*. Such etiological exactitude in the naming of a disease is uncommon because the discovery of the existence of a disease generally precedes by many years the discovery of its cause. In certain instances — that of syphilis, for one — a cure has been found before the cause of the disease has been determined. The causes of numerous familiar ailments, including several of the most malignant, are still unknown. Smallpox, for example, dates back to at least the third century B.C., yet science is still unable to say exactly what causes it or exactly how it is transmitted. The dispatch with which the *Rickettsia* microörganism was identified made it possible to give the disease a definitive name. As a jig-time medical project, the investigation was probably unique. The cause of rickettsialpox and its means of transmission were established just seven months and seven days after its first known victim, an eleven-year-old boy, came down with it on the afternoon of February 23, 1946.

The boy was Edmund Lohr, Jr., the son of Mr. and Mrs. Edmund Lohr, of 141-12 Seventy-eighth Road, in the Kew Gardens section of Queens. Mr. Lohr is the head night auditor of the Shelton Hotel, at Lexington Avenue and Forty-ninth Street. The family occupies a third-floor apartment in an attractive, moderate-priced housing development called Regency Park, which was completed in 1939. Regency Park consists of sixty-three three-story buildings, in which there is a total of five hundred and forty-five more or less identical flats, and covers three large blocks. It is bounded by Union Turnpike, Seventy-eighth Avenue, Main Street, and 141st Street, and it is trisected by Seventy-ninth Avenue and Seventy-eighth Road. The apartment in which the Lohrs live is in the middle block. Mrs. Lohr clearly recollects the start of her son's illness. "Edmund came in from playing, looking sick and grippy," she says. "He said he hurt all over. Well, I put him to bed and took his temperature. It was over a hundred and one, so I telephoned our doctor and he came around as soon as he could. Before he left, he began to look very serious, and I remember he said, 'I've got a case on my hands.' "

The physician who was thus candidly disturbed is Dr. Benjamin Shankman, a young general practitioner with a warm bedside manner, whose office is a block north of Regency Park. He recalls that when he reached the Lohr apartment, Edmund's temperature was a hundred and three. Upon examining the child, Dr. Shankman found a pimple-like lesion on his back and a somewhat swollen gland near the right armpit. He tentatively diagnosed the illness as chicken pox. It was a plausible diagnosis, and it might have stuck if Mrs. Lohr had not pointed out, with reasonable surprise, that Edmund had already *had* chicken pox, some years before. This disclosure naturally unsettled Dr. Shankman, but he sought to reassure himself with the thought that the earlier diagnosis, which had been made by another man, might not have been accurate. There was no getting around the fact, however, that the boy seemed to be a lot sicker than the average chicken-pox sufferer. Dr. Shankman decided that he'd better wait awhile to ascertain if more lesions would develop, and then see.

Two or three days later, there was a generous rash of lesions for Dr. Shankman to study. Careful examination convinced him that they were not precisely like the pox of chicken pox. He therefore discarded the chicken-pox theory and took a blood count. It revealed the presence of a high percentage of white cells, a characteristic of cases of severe infection. Meanwhile, Edmund's temperature was fluctuating eccentrically. At one time, it climbed as high as a hundred and six — a blisteringly high fever, even for a child. Dr. Shankman concluded that his patient had better be put in a hospital, if only for observation. "I was beginning to get scared," he says. Mr. and Mrs. Lohr were even less composed. On February 28th, they and Dr. Shankman took Edmund in a taxi to the Kew Gardens General Hospital, the nearest to their home, where the boy was at first refused admittance, because the examining physician, falling into Dr. Shankman's earlier error, thought that he had chicken pox, and the institution was not equipped to care for patients suffering from a contagious disease. After appealing to several of the authorities there, however, Dr. Shankman succeeded in getting Edmund admitted, and the boy was put to bed in a remote and isolated room. Then Dr. Shankman prescribed a regimen of penicillin therapy. Edmund was given tests for various illnesses during the next few days. The results were all negative. Presently, he began to get well. He was released on March 4th, as good as new. Dr. Shankman closed his record of the case with the cautiously generalized, though not inaccurate, diagnostic notation, "Sepsis, with a rash."

Most physicians recover promptly from the distress of uncertainty. They are accustomed to it. Within a week or so, Dr. Shankman had almost managed to forget his unnerving experience. Then, one morning in the middle of March, having been summoned for what sounded over the telephone like a routine case, he found himself confronted by another unruly fever, with glandular swelling and a small, pimplish lesion. Later, he came to recognize lesions of this nature as an unmistakable symptom of the strange disease. The patient on this occasion was a woman of thirty-four who lived a few doors from the Lohrs. Dr. Shankman's heart sank as he examined her, but also his interest quickened, for he strongly suspected that he was up against the same freakish thing again. He still had no idea of what it was, but he did have a pretty good idea of what it *wasn't*. The tests made on the Lohr boy had shown that it wasn't any of the diseases it most resembled — chicken pox, typhus, endemic typhus, dengue fever, Japanese river fever, Rocky Mountain spotted fever, smallpox, or infectious mononucleosis. Dr. Shankman checked back over his records of the Lohr case and realized that he had no reason to be certain that the penicillin had been responsible for the boy's recovery. This time, therefore, he tried one of the sulfonamides. It seemed to be no more and no less effective than the penicillin. Since the powers of these two drugs are not identical, the Doctor was inclined to suspect that the disease he was confronted with was not affected by either.

This hunch of Dr. Shankman's was strengthened when, before the month was out, another of his Regency Park patients, a middle-aged woman, came down with the same illness. Treated only with aspirin, codeine, and reassuring conversation, she recovered in about the same length of time as the others had. Four or five more cases came to the Doctor's attention during April. They, too, responded favorably to non-medicinal therapy. Dr. Shankman reached the conclusion that the disease was at least self-limiting. Moreover, it appeared to be accompanied by no complications or troublesome aftereffects. "Those were very comforting things to know," he says, "especially as it was beginning to turn up all over the place. Also, people in the neighborhood were naturally getting a little upset about it. It was nice to be able to assure them that it wasn't anything fatal, or even very serious. As a matter of fact, it's been nice to know that ever since, for we have yet to find a cure." At around this time, some residents of Kew Gardens got into the habit of calling the ailment Shankman's disease. Dr. Shankman laughs modestly when he recalls that brief promise of lasting fame. "Well," he says, "I guess I did see all the very first cases." Meanwhile, other Kew Gardens physicians had begun to encounter the same affliction. They were not tempted to call it Shankman's disease. They did, however, tend to agree with him that it was probably something disconcertingly new. Talking with these colleagues and reviewing his records, Dr. Shankman found that the disease was occurring only among residents of Regency Park. That struck him as odd, since there was nothing singular about the place that he could see. There were a dozen new cases in May, still all in Regency Park. Toward the end of that month, Dr. Shankman, feeling that the time had come for official action, reported the existence of the new disease and his perplexities concerning it to the Department of Health, which for a while seemed to show a depressing lack of interest.

As summer came on, more and more cases of rickettsialpox appeared in Regency Park. In spite of the assurances of Dr. Shankman and other physicians that the disease was not dangerous, an understandable apprehension spread through the three blighted blocks. People began to feel trapped.

Several gave up their flats and moved away, preferring the agonies of homehunting to illness. Their apartments did not remain vacant long; there were plenty of other people who evidently preferred the risk of illness to homelessness. Many residents of Regency Park began to experience a kind of social ostracism. Their acquaintances elsewhere in the city, after hearing rumors of the pestilence, hesitated to visit them. "It got so our oldest and best friends would hem and haw and act perfectly hateful when I asked them over to dinner," a woman who was an early victim of the disease remembers. "Why, even my own mother wouldn't come and see me."

Presently, after some intramural fumbling, the Health Department started its own inquiry by sending two of its most expert investigators to Kew Gardens. They interviewed a few of the sick, the convalescent, and the recovered, made some blood tests, conferred inconclusively with the neighborhood doctors, and hospitalized several patients for close, if rather fruitless, examination. Nearly a hundred cases, all among residents of Regency Park, had been reported by then, and the incidence of the disease was nearing epidemic proportions. A few days later, the newspapers got wind of the trouble. On Friday morning, July 19th, the *Times* carried a not entirely unruffled story in which Dr. Shankman was quoted as saying that the illness somewhat resembled Rocky Mountain spotted fever. The following Thursday evening, Dr. Shankman received a telephone call at his office from a man named Charles Pomerantz, who said that he had a theory about what the shriller newspapers had taken to referring to as the "Kew Gardens Mystery Fever," and asked if he could pay the physician a visit. Dr. Shankman had never heard of Mr. Pomerantz, but he told him to come right over, for at that point he was ready to listen to anyone with a fresh approach to the subject. What Mr. Pomerantz, who spoke guardedly, wanted, it turned out, was to inspect the Regency Park basements, and he hoped that Dr. Shankman could arrange it for him. The Doctor encouraged his visitor to be a bit more specific. Then, though more startled than convinced by what Mr. Pomerantz had to say, Dr. Shankman agreed to help. He is thankful that he did.

Mr. Pomerantz, a small, pink-and-white, highly combustible man of fifty who came to this country from Poland at an early age, is the president of the Bell Exterminating Company, on Hudson Street. He is also a gifted, self-taught entomologist, and something of an authority on ticks. He became an exterminator in 1936, after spending nearly twenty remunerative, but spiritually unrewarding, years in the jungles of Seventh Avenue as a manufacturer of ladies' coats. A brother-in-law, David Cantor, at that time a jaded pharmacist, wheedled Mr. Pomerantz into joining him in the exterminating business. "I was unhappy and restless and ripe for almost anything," Mr. Pomerantz says, "but when David suggested we become exterminators, I recoiled. Cockroaches! Bedbugs! Rats! That went against my aesthetic sense. I am a man who keeps a volume of Keats on my bedside table, and I have progressed in fiddle playing to Mendelssohn. But then I thought, 'But pest control is science, and science enjoys a kinship with the arts. Why should I find it more repulsive than ladies' ready-to-wear?' So I assured David I was with him, and we hired a couple of experienced operators." Mr. Pomerantz let his fiddle-playing slide, abandoned Keats, and embarked on a course of technical reading. "It was a challenge to me," he says. "My blood raced with enthusiasm. First, I learned the façade, and finally I began to learn the marrow of the subject. I began to specialize in everything, especially ticks."

When Mr. Pomerantz opened his *Times* on the morning of July 19th and learned what was happening at Regency Park, his blood raced again. "I was intensely fascinated," he says. "Here was a disease resembling Rocky Mountain spotted fever. Rocky Mountain spotted fever is transmitted by the bite of a *tick!* And the tick is my specialty. I said to myself, 'If even the *Herr Doktors* are baffled, then Charles Pomerantz has a moral right to look into it.' " Mr. Pomerantz exercised his moral right on the afternoon of the following day by going out to Regency Park and thoughtfully casing the buildings from the street. He disclosed his identity to no one, not wishing his mission to be suspected of being tainted with commercialism. "I walked and walked," he says, "studying the outside economy, getting the feel of the problem. I asked people I met if many ticks had been found in the neighborhood, but nobody had ever heard of any. Even the owners of two dog kennels just across the street from the south block of apartments told me they had seen no ticks. And yet the disease had appeared in almost every building. With my knowledge of the mechanism and habits of ticks, I found it fantastic to believe that enough ticks — it would take hundreds, thousands — to cause so many people to become ill could suddenly invade an area without anybody finding a single one, not even kennelmen. Ticks are not so small that they are invisible, and when they are gorged with the blood of the necessary host, they are as big as a kidney bean. Besides, New York is not known for anything but the brown dog tick, which is not thought to carry infection to man. A puzzle!" Mr. Pomerantz went home that night as baffled as the doctors.

He was not, however, disheartened. He returned to Regency Park the next day, Sunday, and resumed his sharp-eyed, reflective strolling. Nothing came of it. On Tuesday morning, he trotted back for another look. By that time, he was convinced that the outside economy of the place was immaculate. He prepared to consider the inside economy. "I reasoned that if the cause of the trouble was inside," he says, "then there must be some locomotive mechanism that could go here, there, and everywhere through the buildings, thus spreading the infection. I asked myself, "What is the most obvious such mechanism?' The answer came at once — a rat or mouse. But rats or mice are not known to *transmit* any rash-producing disease. So the rat or the mouse, whichever it is, must be merely the host — or more entomologically, the reservoir — to a disease-bearing parasite that can bite and infect man. I worked the relationship out in my mind. The rat or mouse — and probably the mouse, because I had learned that there were many mice in the buildings but few rats — would be what we call the usual host, with man just the accidental host. But what kind of parasite? Then I had the answer. It flashed into my mind, and I said to myself, 'Ticks out! Mites in!' "

The lack of intense conviction entertained by Dr. Shankman when Mr. Pomerantz presented this hypothesis to him is not surprising. From a medical viewpoint, it was a fairly eccentric notion. Most of the doctors who had treated cases of the peculiar disease were almost certain by then that the characteristic initial lesion was the bite of some minute creature, but they had little reason to suspect mites of being the guilty parties. At the time, it was generally believed that mites could transmit only two serious febrile diseases — Japanese river fever and endemic typhus. Both of these are rarely found in the United States, and anyway both had been eliminated from consideration in this instance by laboratory tests. Moreover, the mouse, unlike the rat, had never been proved to be a reservoir for disease-bearing parasites. Mr. Pomerantz admits that hitting upon the mouse as the probable host was largely intuitive. He is persuaded, however, that in singling out mites as the carriers — or vectors, as such agents are known — of the disease he was guided entirely by deduction.

Mites are insectlike organisms, closely related to ticks. Both are members of the Arachnida, a class that also includes spiders and scorpions. Compared to a tick, a mite is a minute animal. A mite, when fully engorged, is about the size of the strawberry seed. In that state, it is approximately ten times its usual, or unfed, size. So far, science has classified at least thirty families of mites, most of which are vegetarian and indifferent to man and all other animals. The majority of the parasitic, bloodsucking mites have to feed once in every four or five days in order to live. Most mites of this type attach themselves to a host only long enough to engorge, and drop off, replete, after fifteen or twenty minutes. No one ever feels the bite of a mite — or of a tick, either, for that matter — until the animal has dropped off. (Entomologists believe that both creatures, at the instant they bite, excrete a fluid that anesthetizes a small surrounding area of the body of the host.) Mites are only infrequently found in this country and until recently were practically unknown in New York City. Consequently, very few Americans, even physicians and exterminators, have ever seen a mite. Mr. Pomerantz is one of those who have. He came across some in line of duty on three occasions in 1945.

His first encounter was with cheese mites, a nonparasitic variety, in a private house at Hastings-on-Hudson. Some months later, in two widely separated Manhattan apartment buildings, he found infestations of the Oriental rat mite, a suspected vector of endemic typhus. These successive discoveries made a deep impression on Mr. Pomerantz. "Three distinct infestations all of a sudden," he says. "Three warnings that New York and vicinity were no longer immune. I became alerted on mites."

Sponsored by Dr. Shankman, Mr. Pomerantz received permission from the building superintendent at Regency Park to explore the basements of the development on Sunday, July 28th. At one o'clock that afternoon, equipped with a flashlight, a magnifying glass, a couple of two-ounce specimen bottles, and a fine-pointed camel's-hair brush, he ducked resolutely into a cellar on Seventy-ninth Avenue. "I had that Stonewall Jackson feeling," he says. "I *knew* there were mites somewhere in those buildings and I was determined not to go home until I'd found them. Of course. I wasn't a damn fool and didn't just look anywhere. If a detective is looking for a shady character, he looks where it is probable the criminal would hide. I searched the usual haunts of mites. Mites like to be cozy and sandwiched in. Thigmotropism, this instinct is called. So I examined the little cracks in the walls, and especially the tops of the incinerator doors." Mr. Pomerantz had trudged in and out of a dozen basements, and aroused scores of mice, before he spotted his first mite. It was overfed and sluggish, and, using the tip of his brush, he had no trouble flicking it into one of his bottles. By six o'clock, when he knocked off, he had bagged forty-five specimens, some unfed, some bloated. Success had left him shaken. "I, a humble pest-control operator, had found something to relieve the uncertainty of men of scientific learning," he says. "I can't describe my sensation of glory."

Mr. Pomerantz is happily married, but he had not discussed his theory with his wife. He did not do so even now. "There was still a chance that my mites might turn out to be physiologically or morphologically incapable of transmitting such a disease," he says. "I didn't want to raise her false hopes." When Mr. Pomerantz got home, he merely remarked, "Vera, I have something in these bottles that may make medical history." "I don't doubt it," replied Mrs. Pomerantz, a woman in whom, I gathered, the inquisitive instinct is blunted. "Supper is almost ready."

Mr. Pomerantz ate a light supper, read a few chapters of "Medical Entomology," by William B. Herms, and went to bed early. Before he got to sleep, he had decided to take his mites down to Washington the next day and get an authoritative opinion on them from a professional acquaintance, C. F. W. Muesebeck, who is the head of the Division of Insect Identification of the United States Department of Agriculture.

It was midafternoon when Mr. Pomerantz reached Mr. Muesebeck's office. Mr. Muesebeck, after hearing the mite theory, examined the specimens with interest and then dispatched them to one of his colleagues, Dr. E. W. Baker, a mite specialist, for identification. An hour or so later, Dr. Baker reported that the mites were members of a rather rare species, *Allodermanyssus sanguineus,* discovered and classified in Egypt in 1913, and that, although they had no medical history, they had always been looked upon by parasitologists as possible transmitters of disease. Mr. Pomerantz received this stimulating news with a scientist's urbanity.

"But I was all electricity inside," he says. "I was vibrating. I felt wonderful. Mr. Muesebeck even asked me to collect some more specimens for them." Mr. Pomerantz left his mites in the hands of the government and hopped the next train back to New York. That night, he told his wife everything. "You are to be congratulated," he remembers her saying calmly, to which he replied, throbbing with hope and prophecy, "Something has been accomplished, but greater events are coming."

By this time, the more general investigation of the new disease conducted by the city health authorities was well under way. It embraced the clinical, etiological, and epidemiological aspects of the malady. Among those called in to help was a senior assistant surgeon in the United States Public Health Service named Robert J. Huebner. It is customary for municipal authorities to ask the Public Health Service for assistance with troublesome cases. The Service welcomes such invitations, especially because it likes to show what can be accomplished by its National Institute of Health, at Bethesda, Maryland, where it maintains a high-powered staff and superb laboratory facilities. Dr. Huebner, who is young, tough-minded, and carefully unenthusiastic, is a staff worker at the Institute. His assignment in this instance was to try to determine the cause of the disease. He suspected, as did several other investigators, that some member of the genus *Rickettsia* was responsible for the infection. That would account for the resemblance of the disease to Rocky Mountain spotted fever and to typhus, both of which are rickettsial ailments. The rickettsiae, which are named for the late Dr. Howard T. Ricketts, the American pathologist who discovered them, in 1909, are a class of minute bacteria-like organisms, much smaller than real bacteria and generally very elusive. Dr. Huebner buckled down to his job without much expectation of success.

The usual method of isolating a disease organism, and the one that Dr. Huebner followed, involves inoculating a group of highly susceptible laboratory animals whose reactions to disease are known to be similar to man's with a specimen of blood obtained from a person suffering from the disorder. Only if an animal becomes sick and exhibits the symptoms of the disease, as happens with exasperating infrequency in the case of so mild an affliction as rickettsialpox, is the transmission considered a success. The next step is simply a check to make certain that the results of the first were not a fluke. It consists of inoculating another group of animals with a fluid made from diseased brain tissue of the infected animals. If any animals in the second group come down with the disease, the organism is presumed to have been isolated, and fluid made from the brain tissue of these animals is then injected into the yolk sac of a fertile chicken egg. There the organisms multiply with exceptional alacrity, and thus a denser concentration of them is obtained. Smears of the yolk sac are next placed on slides — a very delicate operation — and at last, if everything has gone right, the organisms become visible under the microscope and, with luck, identifiable. For weeks, checking and rechecking in the Institute's laboratories, Dr. Huebner tried in this way to isolate the organism responsible for the Regency Park epidemic. He travelled tirelessly back and forth between Kew Gardens and Bethesda, conferring with Dr. Shankman on the clinical aspects of the illness, procuring new specimens of blood, and supervising the inoculation of hundreds of animals — white rats, cotton rats, rice rats, guinea pigs, rabbits, monkeys, and Syrian hamsters, which are a cross between a rat and a guinea pig. In all, he took specimens of blood from about twenty patients.

Only one specimen turned out to be of a strength sufficient to produce infection in any of the animals. Dr. Huebner had hardly counted on even that. It was obtained, on July 26th — by which time about a hundred and twenty cases of the disease had been reported — from one of Dr. Shankman's many patients, a twenty-two-year-old woman named Marjory Kaplan. Miss Kaplan has since achieved a kind of immortality in medical literature as the donor of what is called, as a rather stark tribute to her, the M.K. Organism. For a while, it looked to Dr. Huebner as if her morbid gift, like those from the other patients, had been made in vain. "Then," he says, "on August 4th, nine days after we had inoculated five mice and two guinea pigs with Miss Kaplan's blood, a fortuitous incident occurred. The guinea pigs and three of the mice hadn't reacted at all to the serum. One of the other mice had reacted, all right, but it had got sick and died at night, when nobody was around. By the time we found it, it was of no use to us. Well, I happened to be standing beside the cage where we were keeping those mice and I noticed that one of them was lying down. Then, all of a sudden, it rolled right over and died. Very obliging. We had the organism transferred from it to another group of animals within fifteen mintues. The test went along very nicely from there on. It was a fine, strong strain, apparently. We were able to keep passing it from one animal to another for weeks and weeks." This was the organism that eventually was isolated and recognized as a rickettsia. Later, several other tests revealed that the organism was a previously unknown species of the genus.

Mr. Pomerantz, in the meantime, had dispatched another

batch of Regency Park mites to the Division of Insect Identification. They, too, were *Allodermanyssus sanguineus*, Mr. Muesebeck reported. He didn't ask for any more, and, feeling a little let down, Mr. Pomerantz returned halfheartedly to exterminating. He couldn't think of anything else to do. Then, on August 16th, he was exhilarated all over again by a telephone call from Dr. Huebner, whose activities he had been wistfully following in the newspapers. Dr. Huebner, it developed, had been informed of Mr. Pomerantz's discovery by Mr. Muesebeck. "It was an interesting piece of information," Dr. Huebner says. "We were beginning to get somewhere in our isolation tests and we knew that Regency Park was crawling with mice, but we didn't know what was actually carrying the organism. Pomerantz's mites sounded like the missing link. If we could produce the disease in a laboratory with mites and then trace its cause back to the same organism, we'd have a very illuminating cycle. Also, if we could definitely establish it as a mouse-borne and mite-transmitted disease, we'd have not only the cause but the preventative as well. It would simply be a matter of keeping down the mouse population." Dr. Huebner's telephone call to Mr. Pomerantz was to ask if he would care to catch some mites for *him*. Mr. Pomerantz didn't have to be urged. That very day, he abandoned his business, for what turned out to be the rest of the summer, and raced out to Regency Park. The next morning, he met Dr. Huebner there and happily handed him a generous sample of mites. His impression of Dr. Huebner was favorable. "I saw he was a true scientist," Mr. Pomerantz says. "He knew how to say, 'I don't know.' We got along fine. I had been afraid that he might think I was a smart alex who was just seeking commercial publicity, but he understood right away that I was as much above reproach as Caesar's wife."

Mr. Pomerantz spent seven weeks in the basements of Regency Park, blissfully gathering mites. Dr. Huebner was insatiable. The days flew by. Occasionally, at Dr. Huebner's suggestion, Mr. Pomerantz varied his work by trapping mice, and to his delight he found most of them to be ridden with disease-carrying mites. Once, he had the satisfaction of capturing a mouse on which ten mites were feeding. Toward the end of August, when Dr. Huebner began to give most of his attention to the mite phase of his study, a field laboratory, staffed by Public Health Service operatives, was set up in the basement of one of the apartment houses, in order to expedite the processing and shipping of Mr. Pomerantz's catches. On September 10th, one of the Service's foremost parasitologists, Dr. William L. Jellison, who is engaged in research at an experimental station at Hamilton, Montana, was called to Regency Park to lend an experienced hand in the conduct of the laboratory. He, too, impressed Mr. Pomerantz as a true scientist. "Dr. Jellison never remembered to eat," Mr. Pomerantz says. "I always had to keep reminding him that we'd missed lunch and that it was now past dinnertime. He subsisted on love of work. I found his attitude very contagious. And yet somehow I gained five pounds."

On the morning of Tuesday, October 1st, Dr. Huebner, who had spent the weekend at Bethesda, sauntered into the basement field laboratory. Mr. Pomerantz was alone in the room. Dr. Huebner grinned at him. "Well, Charlie," he said casually, "we've made it." "Bravo!" Mr. Pomerantz shouted. It was his last utterance for several minutes. "I was suddenly stricken dumb," he says. "I turned pale and weak.

I realized that he had said more than that the investigation was a success. That 'we' included *me!* Dr. Huebner of the United States Public Health Service was calling Charles Pomerantz of the Bell Exterminating Company his scientific colleague. Who can describe my wonderful feelings? It was like meeting Mischa Elman and I had my fiddle and he had his fiddle and we sat down and played together Mendelssohn's Concerto in E minor."

Birds of a Feather

ONE morning toward the end of April, in 1945, Dr. Karl F. Meyer, Director of the George Williams Hooper Foundation for Medical Research, at the University of California, received a somewhat breathless letter from a doctor who introduced himself as an attending physician at the Southampton Hospital, in Suffolk County, Long Island. His name, I'll say, was Cornelius Barton, and his letter was a request for help and counsel. Dr. Barton had a hunch. A few days earlier, he informed Dr. Meyer, he had encountered a case that struck him as uncomfortably provocative. The patient was a handyman on one of the numerous duck farms in that part of the Island, forty-four years old, and white. He had been admitted to the hospital on April 6th, suffering from chills, headache, and abdominal distention, and with a temperature of a hundred and three. Auscultation revealed a slight respiratory rattle. This was presently traced, by a chest X-ray, to a patchy inflammation of the lower right lung. There was, however, no cough, and, as it turned out, no further pulmonary involvement. After three days, during which treatment was confined to bed rest and small doses of sulfadiazine, his temperature dropped, his chest cleared, and he was discharged to convalesce at home. He was now pretty well recovered. Having thus delivered himself of the pertinent facts, Dr. Barton moved on to speculation. The general nature of the case, of course, presented no great diagnostic challenge. It was almost certainly an atypical, or virus, pneumonia. Ordinarily, he would have been inclined to let it go at that. But this, he felt, was not an ordinary case. He had been inspired to attempt a more definitive reading. The trouble was he lacked the experience and the laboratory facilities to put it to a test. Dr. Meyer, he knew, possessed an abundance of both. Dr. Barton had on hand a sample of blood extracted from his patient on the third day of illness. Might he send it to him? He would like to have it examined by the complement-fixation method for evidence of ornithotic pneumonitis. Unless he was badly mistaken, he had just discovered a case of psittacosis acquired from a barnyard duck.

Dr. Barton's choice of a collaborator, though awkwardly transcontinental, was anything but arbitrary. It was practically unavoidable. Dr. Meyer is not merely the outstanding authority in this country on the ecology and epidemiology of psittacosis but back in 1945 he was almost the only one. The excitement that animated Dr. Barton's appeal was also natural enough. Psittacosis is parrot fever. At that time, its transmission was thought to be largely, if not altogether, confined to birds of the psittacine group. This includes such parrots as Amazons, African grays, cockatoos, macaws, parakeets, lovebirds, and lories. Although all psittacines are potential reservoirs of psittacosis, most outbreaks of the disease in man have been caused by either parrots or parakeets. Psittacosis was recognized as an entity of avian origin by Jacob Ritter, a perceptive Swiss pathologist, in 1879. His portrait of its clinical manifestations, which he observed in a family of seven whose misfortune it had been to acquire an infected parrot, is still considered a generally excellent likeness. Ritter called his discovery "pneumotyphus." Its present name, which derives from *psittakos*, the Greek for "parrot," was suggested in 1895 by a French physician named Antonin Morange.

Until 1929, psittacosis was universally regarded as among the rarest of rare diseases. In that year, a pandemic of almost global proportions rendered this agreeable assumption abruptly and permanently infirm. It began in Córdoba, in the Argentine, shortly after the opening of an auction, attended by dealers from all over the world, of several thousand Brazilian parrots and other psittacine birds. That was around the middle of July. By August, the disease had spread to Tucumán, a city in a neighboring province. The following month, it exploded in Buenos Aires. Among its first victims there were twelve actors in a new play whose cast also contained a parrot. Two of them, and the parrot, died. The epidemic next appeared in Switzerland — in Geneva, where it was soon traced to a number of sickly psittacines recently imported from Córdoba. During November and December, outbreaks of similar origin flared up in a dozen German cities and in Warsaw, Prague, and Vienna. Early in 1930, the disease was everywhere in Europe — Denmark, Holland, France, England, Spain, Portugal, Italy — as well as in Algeria, in Egypt, and in the Middle East. It reached Canada and the United States during the winter of 1929–30, striking first, and almost simultaneously, in Philadelphia, in Providence, and in Warren, Ohio. By midsummer, a total of nearly two hundred cases, with thirty-three deaths, had been reported in fifteen states. The last outbreak usually included in the pandemic occurred in October, 1930, in Hawaii. Exactly how many people were stricken in the course of those fifteen months has never been determined, and estimates vary widely. The most conservative put the number at approximately eight hundred. Probably, considering the unfamiliarity of the disease and the ambiguity of its symptoms, it was at least twice that. The number of fatal cases is less uncertain. There were, roughly, a hundred and fifty.

The pandemic had two immediate results. One, as might be expected, was a salubrious quickening of interest among medical scientists in the anatomy of psittacosis. Their efforts were richly and rapidly productive. By the end of 1931, its cause had been found, its mechanics charted, and Ritter's description of its salient signs revised for modern readers. Since then, though at a somewhat less headlong pace, many of its remaining riddles have been fathomed with equal thoroughness. The agent responsible for psittacosis is a filterable organism intermediate in size between a virus and a bacillus, but most authorities find it convenient to call it a virus. Fortunately, it has all the few redeeming weaknesses of both of its nearest relatives. It is vulnerable to most antibiotics, it confers on its surviving victims a more or less prolonged resistance to reinfection, and it is incapable of growth and reproduction outside the body of a living animal host. The communicability of psittacosis is also providentially peculiar. Although the organism is readily airborne and enters the body by way of the upper respiratory tract, its passage from one human being to another is almost unheard of; it has been reported just thirty times. To the best of medical knowledge, the only significant source of infection to man is dust heavily and freshly contaminated with the droppings of a psittacotic bird.

The other immediate result of the 1929–30 pandemic was the establishment by the affected nations of public-health regulations designed to prevent its recurrence. Those set up in the United States were among the most stringent. They included a federal embargo on all alien psittacines for commercial resale, restrictions largely prohibiting the interstate transportation of any members of the family, and an elaborate network of supplementary defenses devised by the various states. The majority of the regulations became effective early in 1930. Early in 1952, the embargo on imports was substantially modified and practically all the other regulations were rescinded. This action, though abrupt, was in no sense impulsive. It was, if anything, deliberate to the point of procrastination. Since the end of 1945, it had been abundantly plain that as a means of ridding the country of psittacosis the regulations were totally ineffectual. The disease is ineradicably here, and probably has been for years.

Dr. Meyer's reply to Dr. Barton's request was composed on Thursday, April 26th. It was delivered the following Monday. Dr. Barton found it on his desk when he came in at about five from a round of afternoon calls. "This is in reply to your letter of April 16th," Dr. Meyer wrote. "I want to tell you first that I will be only too glad to examine the blood serum of the patient who is now suffering from an atypical pneumonia which you suspect to be connected epidemiologically with Pekin ducks. In case we prove this pneumonia to be caused by the ornithosis or psittacosis agents, some steps should then be taken to test the blood serum of the Pekin ducks. Until relatively recently, only the representatives of the parrot family were suspected of being the hosts of ornithosis or psittacosis virus. With the discovery that the infection occurs quite extensively in pigeons . . . and also in seagulls, I see no reasons why the Pekin ducks should not be the hosts of a similar or identical virus. Recently, I had a letter from Philadelphia with a history of a man who was exposed to wild ducks. This serum gave a strongly positive reaction for the ornithosis virus. Therefore, the reasonableness that he became infected by handling ducks is great. . . . Any time you wish to send the sera, please do so. . . . Preferably, two samples should be sent — one collected during the first few days of the illness and another one between the fifteenth and twentieth days of convalescence. We have shown that penicillin is quite effective in the treatment of these infections. Ordinarily, we use a dosage of 20,000 units every three hours during the first forty-eight hours, and then reduce the dosage to ten. . . ."

"I don't know what kind of an answer I expected," Dr. Barton says. "But you may be sure it was nothing like that. Not even in my most hopeful moments. About all I really asked at that point was to be taken seriously. I didn't see how Dr. Meyer could turn me down. Not completely. Still, I can't deny that the possibility had occurred to me. And I knew if he did I was sunk. Just another general practitioner who had made a fool of himself. I was pretty sure I hadn't, but I could have, of course. Very easily. I knew next to nothing about ornithology, and not much more about psittacosis. I'd seen only one confirmed case in my life. That was back in 1930, at medical school, and he was dead. I sat in on a post-mortem. Apart from a little reading, that was the extent of my knowledge. So far as I can recall, I never even thought of psittacosis again until that day in 1945. There was no occasion to. Why I happened to think of it then is hard to say. Psittacosis is a form of pneumonitis, and I was quite certain that my patient — Haupt was his name — had a pneumonitis, but pneumonitis doesn't necessarily mean psittacosis. Hardly. All I knew was that in Haupt's case I thought it did. And when I began to look around for a possible source of infection, the only birds in sight were ducks. There are some things you just can't explain. Something happens and your mind begins to percolate, and sometimes something comes out. Well, I thought this was one of those times. And Dr. Meyer agreed. At least, that was the impression I got. He isn't the type to get excited over trivialities. But his letter was a good deal more than encouraging. It was also most instructive. I think I knew that the virus had been demonstrated in pigeons and gulls. Vaguely. I had no idea how extensively, though, and, of course, the wild-duck angle was something altogether new. So was the tip on penicillin. Penicillin was still a good deal of an unknown quantity back in those days. Nobody was exactly sure what it could and couldn't do. When I came to that passage, I stopped and stared. Nothing could have been more opportune. Because over the weekend I'd come across what looked like two more cases of the same. They were a white man and a colored woman, both duck-farm people, and both sicker than Haupt ever was. And neither one had shown the slightest response to sulfadiazine.

"Well, Dr. Meyer's word was good enough for me. I trotted up to the wards and went right to work. To make up for lost time, I started out with twenty-five thousand units for each. If that didn't do the job, I was prepared to go even higher. I won't say I was really worried. Neither one of them appeared to be in serious trouble. But you never know. I also took the precaution of arranging for a couple of samples of blood. However, Haupt was first on the list. I got a second specimen of his blood in the morning. He was a little past the twentieth day of convalescence, but I couldn't help that. At any rate, my package was on its way to Dr. Meyer by noon, air-mail special delivery. That was on Tuesday, May 1st. Then I waited. Or tried to. Until Sunday. On Sunday morning, as I sat down to breakfast, the telephone rang. It was Western Union with a wire from Dr. Meyer. The message read: 'SERUM PATIENT HAUPT FIXES COMPLEMENT WITH PSITTACOSIS ANTIGEN IN DILUTION ONE TO THIRTY-TWO. REACTION DIAGNOSTICALLY POSITIVE. PLEASE SEND SERA FROM SICK DUCKS.'

"So I was right. Or perhaps it would be more accurate to say I wasn't wrong. A ratio of one to thirty-two is unequivocal. In view of the other clinical findings, it meant that Haupt had very definitely suffered an attack of psittacosis. Which was extremely gratifying. But, of course, that's all it did mean. It merely confirmed the existence of a psittacosis problem. It didn't tell us where he got his infection. The real point at issue remained to be proved. My idea that the ducks were the source of the trouble was still just a notion. Unless we could show that the ducks were infected, I obviously hadn't accomplished very much. Well, there are two procedures by which the presence of the psittacosis virus can be demonstrated in a bird. One is the blood-serum, or complement-fixation, test. The other is rather more complicated. It works something like this. A group of laboratory mice are inoculated with material obtained from the vital organs of the suspected host. Presently, if all goes well, the mice become sick and die. An autopsy is then performed and the spleen removed for microscopic examination. The result, when successful, is isolation of the organism. But it isn't always that simple. It's often necessary to make another passage to a second group of mice. In any event, it takes from two weeks to a month. Dr. Meyer preferred to start with the blood test. That was understandable. It isn't quite as satisfactory as the other — or at least not with birds. Nevertheless, as a preliminary check, it could save a lot of time and effort. It also made things a bit easier for me. I didn't have to cut up any ducks. Although even getting a few cc.s of duck serum wasn't exactly easy. I had to do a little persuading before the owner of the farm where Haupt had worked finally gave in and let me proceed. He didn't like the implications. In the end, I managed to bleed three birds. The samples reached Dr. Meyer on May 11th. Ten days later, on May 21st, I got his report. He had tested all three samples with every available antigen. The results were uniformly negative.

"That was pretty bitter. I won't say I was surprised. In a way, I'd even expected it. But you know how it is — you can't help hoping. The only consolation was that the findings were essentially inconclusive. A positive reaction — even one — would have been immensely significant. On the other hand, a negative report meant almost nothing. Approximately six million Pekin ducks are grown on Long Island every year. Haupt's employer alone raises several hundred thousand. And we'd examined three. As Dr. Meyer remarked in his report, that hardly constituted a fair test of my hypothesis. He had never supposed that a majority of the ducks might be infected. Possibly, he said, no more than five or ten per cent. A much larger sampling would have to be tested and proved negative before he would be willing to accept the present findings. Of course, all that more or less went without saying, but it helped to hear him say it. I needed all the encouragement I could get. Not just because I'd had high hopes of those samples. I had other worries. My two new patients had responded beautifully to penicillin. In fact, the woman had already gone back home. But the day she left, another case came in. A few days later, another arrived. And he was followed by a third. They were all exactly alike. Sex: Male. Occupation: Duck farmer. Diagnosis: Atypical pneumonia. As it happened, they weren't my cases. I only saw them. But that was enough to take all the joy out of life. In other words, unless Haupt had completely led me astray, we were up against something that looked unpleasantly like an epidemic.

"He hadn't. Dr. Meyer disposed of that possibility, if it was one, very promptly. All he needed was five specimens of blood. I didn't wait to be asked. As a matter of fact, I'd sent them off, along with a full history of each patient, even before I got his report on the ducks. His answer came through on the twenty-eighth. Haupt had plenty of company. Of the five, two — cases 1 and 2 — were definitely positive for psittacosis. No. 3 was probable. The two most recent cases — 4 and 5 — were uncertain. It was simply too early to tell. He suggested I bleed them again. He also asked for another sampling of duck sera. Then he gave me rather a start, for he added that he was sending a copy of this letter to Dr. Robert F. Korns, the acting director of the Division of Communicable Diseases of the New York State Department of Health, at Albany, with a recommendation that the state institute a thorough epidemiological investigation of the matter. I don't know why that should have surprised me — it was certainly the logical next step — but it did. It just hadn't occurred to me, I guess, that I had stumbled onto anything quite that big. It was a little hard to believe."

Dr. Meyer's letter had much the same effect on Dr. Korns. He, too, though for somewhat different reasons, read it with rather a start. Also, like Dr. Barton, he found it a little hard to believe. "I was acquainted with Dr. Meyer," Dr. Korns says. "We'd had some correspondence about something or other a couple of years before. That probably explains why he chose me instead of the State Commissioner. Not, of course, that Dr. Meyer ever needs an introduction. His interest is always welcome. I must say, however, it was a most unusual letter. And a most disturbing one. I don't mean to imply that I was under the impression that psittacosis had been legislated out of existence. None of us had any illusions about that. We saw a few cases — four or five or so — every year. In fact, I even knew that one had recently turned up on Long Island. Psittacosis, being at least nominally communicable, is a reportable disease, and when Dr. Barton got the laboratory report on Haupt, he immediately notified the Suffolk County authorities. Suffolk County is a semi-autonomous unit, but we keep in touch with each other, and they sent us a memo. I read it and dropped it in the file, and that was that. Then I got Dr. Meyer's letter. An occasional case of psittacosis was one thing. But six was quite another. Even without several million ducks in the background. All I could think of was 1930.

"To tell the truth, I had my doubts about the ducks. With all due respect for Dr. Meyer's opinion, I couldn't see that they were necessarily the focus of infection. He seemed to consider it probable. His letter to me contained an explanatory note saying, 'There is every likelihood that an ornithosis problem exists on the duck farms.' That struck me as a trifle strong. The evidence, as far as I could make out, was altogether circumstantial. It could be the ducks. Or it could be something else — gulls, perhaps, or pigeons. Chickens, even. If parrots were out, as they unquestionably were, almost anything was possible. The field was wide open. One thing, however, was sure. Something very strange was happening down on eastern Long Island, and it was up to the state health authorities to do something about it. First of all, though, I wanted to see for myself. Even a routine investigation takes a certain amount of planning. And this one looked like anything but that. A couple of days at the scene did nothing to change my mind. I drove down on Thursday morning, May 31st, stayed over Friday, and came back late Saturday night. My first stop was Riverhead, the Suffolk County seat, where I had a word with the county health commissioner — in those days a man named Davis — and arranged for what help he could give us. As I'd expected, that was mostly good will. The war had practically emptied his office. Then I looked up Dr. Barton, and he introduced me around the Southampton Hospital. I met the staff and I saw the patients and I spent an hour or so with the files. By the time I got back to Albany, I felt a little better. That isn't to say the problem looked any less formidable than it had before. I knew we were in for a long, hard pull. But the outbreak itself wasn't as bad as I had feared. There hadn't been a new case in a week or more. The total — confirmed, probable, and suspected — was still six. There might be more to come, but at least it wasn't an explosion. The clinical picture was also most reassuring. So far, not a single really serious case had turned up.

"I left Dr. Barton with the impression that our investigation would probably begin sometime the following week. That would have been the normal procedure. Unfortunately, it didn't turn out that way. We ran into a series of emergencies — outbreaks of one kind or another that demanded immediate attention — and June was gone before I could spare a man. The war had us all cut down to the bone. We finally got started on the tenth of July. I say 'we,' but actually, except for a few hasty visits, I spent all my time at my desk. Most of the work in the field was handled by an epidemiologist named Donald Tulloch — he's dead now, poor fellow. An extremely able man. He had to be for this particular job. About the only person whose help he could consistently count on was Dr. Barton. The rest of us came and went. Before Tulloch took off for Suffolk County, we had a little conference. It wasn't a very cheerful meeting. The longer we looked at the problem, the bigger it got. Bigger and broader and more complicated. I'd had a peculiar feeling about it ever since I got back from Long Island. But it wasn't until then that I began to understand why. Most epidemiological problems involve just one basic question. This one was different. It involved two. Six people in Suffolk County — they had all been confirmed by then — had psittacosis. Where did they get it? That was one question. The other was this: It was also a fact that those people lived and worked miles away from each other. That meant that the focus of infection was pretty widespread. So why were there only six cases? Six were plenty. But sixty would have been easier to explain.

"I didn't hear from Tulloch for more than a week. Then, on July 18th, he sent in a rough preliminary report. He had been to the hospital, he had talked to half the doctors in the county, and he had done a lot of digging on his own. The result was twelve more cases. All, like the first ones, were more or less mild. There was no question about the diagnosis. In each case, Dr. Meyer had confirmed it by the complement-fixation test. That brought the total up to eighteen. As it happened, not all of that was news to me. I'd had some inkling that the count was rising. I forget from whom — Dr. Barton, probably. He'd called me a couple of times. What *was* news, though, was that only ten of the new cases were duck-farm people. The other two had no connection with ducks at all. One was a section hand on the Long Island Railroad and the other a man who ran a butcher shop in Riverhead. But they both kept chickens, and the section hand's next-door neighbor owned a large flock of pigeons. That added to the confusion with a vengeance. It not only weakened the chain of circumstantial evidence that seemed to implicate the ducks but it also gave us a prominent new suspect. The butcher and the railroad man weren't the only chicken raisers among the whole eighteen victims. Ten of the others were, too. Moreover, just to snarl things up a little more, one of the new patients and one of the original six told Tulloch that they sometimes amused themselves by feeding wild pigeons. A nice mess.

"The rest of the report was an account of work in progress. In spite of the butcher and the railroad man and the chickens, the bulk of the evidence still pointed to the ducks — or, rather, it appeared to. Most of the patients were duck people. But then, so was almost everybody else in that part of Long Island. Any disease in that area would be bound to show a high incidence among people who had something to do with ducks. In other words, was there a real relationship between the farms and the outbreak? Or was it merely fortuitous? Well, Tulloch was doing what he could to find out. His approach was conventional. Exposure to the psittacosis virus may not always cause illness. That's true, of course, of all communicable diseases. It does, however, almost always cause certain relatively permanent changes in the blood — the development of immunizing substances called antibodies — and they can be detected by the complement-fixation test. Tulloch reasoned that if the ducks were the source of the trouble, the blood of all — or at any rate many — of the other farmers would contain evidence of past infection. And the blood of people having no contact with ducks would be normal. He had already bled twelve apparently healthy men and women who worked on one or another of the implicated farms. He was now in the process of selecting a dozen people from the general population in the epidemic area to serve as controls. Both sets of specimens would be in Dr. Meyer's hands by the middle of the following week. Our next move in that phase of the investigation depended entirely upon the laboratory.

"Toward the end of the month, Tulloch came in from the field for a couple of days to attend to some personal matter. He was still around when Dr. Meyer's report arrived. That was Monday morning, July 30th. The results were not exactly what we had expected. Or hoped for. Seven out of the twelve farmers gave positive reactions. But so did three of the controls. Tulloch was at a loss. It seemed to confirm our idea that the focus was pretty widespread. Beyond that, he didn't know what to think. Neither did I. Except that a new and larger sampling was very much in order. Large enough to eliminate any possible distortion. I suggested another series from the implicated farms, one from farms where no cases had occurred, one from a farm where only chickens were raised, and, naturally, a much larger group of controls. Then we might be able to draw some definite conclusions. I also suggested that he hop right to it. Tulloch didn't need any urging. He left immediately after lunch.

"Tuesday morning, with one of the local doctors for a guide, Tulloch started in. They began with the farms. Their first stop was a big establishment near Center Moriches, in the heart of the duck-growing area. I don't believe any of us were quite prepared for what happened next. We should have been, perhaps, but we weren't. What happened was the owner stopped them at the gate. He was pleasant enough, Tulloch told me later, but very firm. There wasn't going to be any bleeding on his place. Or on any other, he hoped. What were we trying to do — put them all out of business? Everybody in the neighborhood was talking about what they called duck fever. The workers were getting scared. A little more investigating and they'd all up and quit. And not only that. If the duck-fever gossip ever reached the market, there wouldn't be any more market. Nobody would even dream of eating another Long Island duck. That, of course, was plain silly. The psittacosis organism enters the body through the respiratory system, not the alimentary canal. Besides, the virus is extremely delicate and couldn't possibly survive the processing that a duck goes through before it reaches the market. Well, Tulloch told him all that and a good deal more, but the answer was still no. It was also no at the next farm. And the next. Then he gave up.

"I got wind of the trouble around noon. One of the big operators, a sort of spokesman for the industry, telephoned our district office in Manhattan and made a formal complaint, and they passed the word along to me. I passed it on to Tulloch. He was in Dr. Barton's office when I finally reached him. The answer, we agreed, was to hold a meeting with some of the leading growers. I was confident that if he could get them to sit down and listen to what we were doing and why, most of them would come around. The only alternative was force. But that kind of coöperation is never very satisfactory. Fortunately, we very seldom have to go that far. Reason usually prevails. And it did in this case. With the help of Dr. Barton and a couple of others, Tulloch rounded up eight or ten of the leaders and they agreed to meet him that night at somebody's house in Eastport. It was a ticklish situation. The growers were dead wrong. Still, you couldn't help but sympathize with them. They were in a tough spot. Tulloch handled it beautifully. He didn't try to argue, he simply stated the problem. Did they want the truth? Or did they prefer gossip and guesses and rumors? Then he left the room and let them decide for themselves. He must have bewitched them. When they called him back, the battle was more than won. They hadn't just withdrawn the complaint and agreed to coöperate. They had even voted to invite him to address the fall meeting of the Long Island Duck Growers Association. From then on, with the growers all behind him, Tulloch made good time. He ended up, on August 10th, with a total of sixty-six new samples. Thirty-three were taken from duck people in various parts of the area. The rest, including two chicken raisers, were all controls. If that didn't clarify the picture a bit, it was hard to say what would.

"Meanwhile, during the past few weeks, I'd had several letters from Dr. Meyer. His confidence in the ducks was still unshaken, but he had finally given up hope of ever proving anything by testing samples of their sera. None of the numerous samples that Dr. Barton had sent him had shown even a faintly positive reaction. So the time had come to try to isolate the organism from tissue. Would we please supply him with the necessary specimens for laboratory testing on mice? Well, we already had — a few, at any rate. Whenever Tulloch or Dr. Barton could either of them find the time. But now that Tulloch had wound up his serological survey, we could settle down in earnest. Dr. Barton let his practice practically drop. The only thing that really interested him any more was psittacosis, and by then the active phase of the outbreak was over. Long over. The last case was No 12 in the group that Tulloch reported in July. Which was a great relief. Keeping Dr. Meyer supplied with material turned out to be a very big job. He wanted plenty and he wanted everything. Not just ducks — although, of course, they were his main concern — but also chickens, pigeons, gulls, crows, and even starlings. I went down myself for a couple of days to help get the project started. We opened up on Monday morning, August 13th, in an old barn on the outskirts of Riverhead. That was headquarters. We killed, autopsied, and prepared all our specimens there. And packed them for shipping. Shipping was the biggest headache of all. The psittacosis organism is extraordinarily fragile. Everything we sent off had to be frozen and packed in dry ice — enough of it to guarantee safe arrival some three thousand miles away, in August. Not all the first few samples made it. It was pretty discouraging. And the first few reports — on a couple of ducks and a pigeon, I think, that Dr. Barton had sent off back in July — did nothing to cheer us up. Negative, one and all. Toward the end of the month, Dr. Meyer sent one of his technicians, Dr. Bernice Eddie, on from the Coast to lend us a hand, and a few days later wrote that he himself was coming East sometime in September, and planned to pay us a visit. Those were about the only pleasant things I remember about the whole of August. Everything else was hard work and hard luck. And then, just after Labor Day, the report on Tulloch's bloods came through. It didn't bear much resemblance to the report on his first survey. Of the thirty-three controls, only two were definitely positive. The balance, or well over ninety per cent of the group, were either completely negative or inconclusive. Among the duck farmers, on the other hand, eight, or twenty-five per cent, were positive. And unmistakably so. Of course, that wasn't final proof. Not by any means. Those two positive controls — to say nothing of the three in the other series — meant that we still had a long way to go. But it was no longer possible to seriously doubt that the ducks were in the picture. They almost had to be.

"They were. Only, it turned out to be quite a sizable picture. And it took a good many weeks to piece it all together. Dr. Meyer had been to New York and out to Riverhead to see our plant and back in California for some little while before his laboratory tests turned up the first organism. The date was Tuesday, October 2nd. It came, very suitably, from the liver of a bird that was born and raised on the farm where Haupt had worked — a three-week-old drake. That cemented the duck as a carrier. But he was just the beginning. By the time we heard about him, there were more. And the news got bigger and bigger. On October 8th, two pigeons came through. Beautifully. Then a lot more ducks and a couple of gulls and a crow. In the end, around the first of November, when we closed up shop, the only bird that hadn't yielded was the starling. Which proved nothing. We hadn't made a really serious effort with starlings. I've forgotten the final score — we got forty or fifty positives from ducks alone — but I remember the estimates we eventually worked out on incidence. They tell the story well enough. Pigeons, we concluded, are the worst. Fifty per cent of them are infected. Gulls come next — forty per cent. Then ducks — thirty-three per cent. The others — chickens and crows — average about twenty. I say estimates. That's what they were at first. Now they're practically facts. Since 1945, there have been a number of other surveys. Every one of them has fully confirmed our conclusions. Psittacosis isn't peculiar to the ducks and gulls and pigeons and chickens and crows of Long Island. It's an endemic disease that may well appear in any bird anywhere.

"For us, isolation of the virus was the grand finale. But it didn't completely wrap things up. There were still a couple of problems. Diagnosis isn't a remedy. What, for example, were we going to do about the situation? Or, rather, what could we do? Well, the answer to that turned out to be wonderfully simple. Nothing. There wasn't anything we could do. Unless, of course, we killed off all the birds on Long Island. And kept them killed off. That may sound more like a rationalization than a solution. Actually, though, there was no great need to do anything. Then or since. The Long Island experience didn't merely broaden our understanding of the potential sources of psittacosis. It also broadened our understanding of the disease itself. We used to think of psittacosis as a pretty serious affair. That was natural. The serious cases were about the only ones we ever saw. Now, I think, it's generally agreed that severe attacks are really rather uncommon. The average victim, as Tulloch's survey very clearly suggested, doesn't even know he's sick. The other problem wasn't really a problem. It was just a loose end — something we wondered about. The cause of the trouble was obviously deeply rooted. Then why did the outbreak happen when it did? Why 1945? Instead of 1944, say, or 1943? We got the answer to that the following year, when there was another little flurry on the farms. So the chances are that 1945 wasn't the first year that part of Long Island had an outbreak of psittacosis. It's probably been going on for generations. Except that in 1945 there was Dr. Barton. And he opened his eyes and saw it."

Sodium Nitrite

Eleven Blue Men

AT about eight o'clock on Monday morning, September 25, 1944, a ragged, aimless old man of eighty-two collapsed on the sidewalk on Dey Street, near the Hudson Terminal. Innumerable people must have noticed him, but he lay there alone for several minutes, dazed, doubled up with abdominal cramps, and in an agony of retching. Then a policeman came along. Until the policeman bent over the old man, he may have supposed that he had just a sick drunk on his hands; wanderers dropped by drink are common in that part of town in the early morning. It was not an opinion that he could have held for long. The old man's nose, lips, ears, and fingers were sky-blue. The policeman went to a telephone and put in an ambulance call to Beekman-Downtown Hospital, half a dozen blocks away. The old man was carried into the emergency room there at eight-thirty. By that time, he was unconscious and the blueness had spread over a large part of his body. The examining physician attributed the old man's morbid color to cyanosis, a condition that usually results from an insufficient supply of oxygen in the blood, and also noted that he was diarrheic and in a severe state of shock. The course of treatment prescribed by the doctor was conventional. It included an instant gastric lavage, heart stimulants, bed rest, and oxygen therapy. Presently, the old man recovered an encouraging, if painful, consciousness and demanded, irascibly and in the name of God, to know what had happened to him. It was a question that, at the moment, nobody could answer with much confidence.

For the immediate record, the doctor made a free-hand diagnosis of carbon-monoxide poisoning — from what source, whether an automobile or a gas pipe, it was, of course, pointless even to guess. Then, because an isolated instance of gas poisoning is something of a rarity in a section of the city as crammed with human beings as downtown Manhattan, he and his colleagues in the emergency room braced themselves for at least a couple more victims. Their foresight was promptly and generously rewarded. A second man was rolled in at ten-twenty-five. Forty minutes later, an ambulance drove up with three more men. At eleven-twenty, two others were brought in. An additional two arrived during the next fifteen minutes. Around noon, still another was admitted. All of these nine men were also elderly and dilapidated, all had been in misery for at least an hour, and all were rigid, cyanotic, and in a state of shock. The entire body of one, a bony, seventy-three-year-old consumptive named John Mitchell, was blue. Five of the nine, including Mitchell, had been stricken in the Globe Hotel, a sunless, upstairs flophouse at 190 Park Row, and two in a similar place, called the Star Hotel, at 3 James Street. Another had been found slumped in the doorway of a condemned building on Park Row, not far from City Hall Park, by a policeman. The ninth had keeled over in front of the Eclipse Cafeteria, at 6 Chatham Square. At a quarter to seven that evening, one more aged blue man was brought in. He had been lying, too sick to ask for help, on his cot in a cubicle in the Lion Hotel, another flophouse, at 26 Bowery, since ten o'clock that morning. A clerk had finally looked in and seen him.

By the time this last blue man arrived at the hospital, an investigation of the case by the Department of Health, to which all outbreaks of an epidemiological nature must be reported, had been under way for five hours. Its findings thus far had not been illuminating. The investigation was conducted by two men. One was the Health Department's chief epidemiologist, Dr. Morris Greenberg, a small, fragile, reflective man of fifty-seven, who is now acting director of the Bureau of Preventable Diseases; the other was Dr. Ottavio Pellitteri, a field epidemiologist, who, since 1946, has been administrative medical inspector for the Bureau. He is thirty-six years old, pale, and stocky, and has a bristling black mustache. One day, when I was in Dr. Greenberg's office, he and Dr. Pellitteri told me about the case. Their recollection of it is, understandably, vivid. The derelicts were the victims of a type of poisoning so rare that only ten previous outbreaks of it had been recorded in medical literature. Of these, two were in the United States and two in Germany; the others had been reported in France, England, Switzerland, Algeria, Australia, and India. Up to September 25, 1944, the largest number of people stricken in a single outbreak was four. That was in Algeria, in 1926.

The Beekman-Downtown Hospital telephoned a report of the occurrence to the Health Department just before noon. As is customary, copies of the report were sent to all the Department's administrative officers. "Mine was on my desk when I got back from lunch," Dr. Greenberg said to me. "It didn't sound like much. Nine persons believed to be suffering from carbon-monoxide poisoning had been admitted during the morning, and all of them said that they had eaten breakfast at the Eclipse Cafeteria, at 6 Chatham Square. Still, it was a job for us. I checked with the clerk who handles assignments and found that Pellitteri had gone out on it. That was all I wanted to know. If it amounted to anything, I knew he'd phone me before making a written report. That's an arrangement we have here. Well, a couple of hours later I got a call from him. My interest perked right up."

"I was at the hospital," Dr. Pellitteri told me, "and I'd talked to the staff and most of the men. There were ten of them by then, of course. They were sick as dogs, but only one was in really bad shape."

"That was John Mitchell," Dr. Greenberg put in. "He died the next night. I understand his condition was hopeless from the start. The others, including the old boy who came in last, pulled through all right. Excuse me, Ottavio, but I just thought I'd get that out of the way. Go on."

Dr. Pellitteri nodded. "I wasn't at all convinced that it was gas poisoning," he continued. "The staff was beginning to doubt it, too. The symptoms weren't quite right. There didn't seem to be any of the headache and general dopiness that you get with gas. What really made me suspicious was this: Only two or three of the men had eaten breakfast in the cafeteria at the same time. They had straggled in all the way from seven o'clock to ten. That meant that the place would have had to be full of gas for at least three hours, which is preposterous. It also indicated that we ought to have had a lot more sick people than we did. Those Chatham Square eating places have a big turnover. Well, to make sure, I checked with Bellevue, Gouverneur, St. Vincent's, and the other downtown hospitals. None of them had seen a trace of cyanosis. Then I talked to the sick men some more.

I learned two interesting things. One was that they had all got sick right after eating. Within thirty minutes. The other was that all but one had eaten oatmeal, rolls, and coffee. He ate just oatmeal. When ten men eat the same thing in the same place on the same day and then all come down with the same illness . . . I told Greenberg that my hunch was food poisoning."

"I was willing to rule out gas," Dr. Greenberg said. A folder containing data on the case lay on the desk before him. He lifted the cover thoughtfully, then let it drop. "And I agreed that the oatmeal sounded pretty suspicious. That was as far as I was willing to go. Common, ordinary, everyday food poisoning — I gathered that was what Pellitteri had in mind — wasn't a very satisfying answer. For one thing, cyanosis is hardly symptomatic of that. On the other hand, diarrhea and severe vomiting are, almost invariably. But they weren't in the clinical picture, I found, except in two or three of the cases. Moreover, the incubation periods — the time lapse between eating and illness — were extremely short. As you probably know, most food poisoning is caused by eating something that has been contaminated by bacteria. The usual offenders are the staphylococci — they're mostly responsible for boils and skin infections and so on — and the salmonella. The latter are related to the typhoid organism. In a staphylococcus case, the first symptoms rarely develop in under two hours. Often, it's closer to five. The incubation period in the other ranges from twelve to thirty-six hours. But here we were with something that hit in thirty minutes or less. Why, one of the men had got only as far as the sidewalk in front of the cafeteria before he was knocked out. Another fact that Pellitteri had dug up struck me as very significant. All of the men told him that the illness had come on with extraordinary suddenness. One minute they were feeling fine, and the next minute they were practically helpless. That was another point against the ordinary food-poisoning theory. Its onset is never that fast. Well, that suddenness began to look like a lead. It led me to suspect that some drug might be to blame. A quick and sudden reaction is characteristic of a great many drugs. So is the combination of cyanosis and shock."

"None of the men were on dope," Dr. Pellitteri said. "I told Greenberg I was sure of that. Their pleasure was booze."

"That was O.K.," Dr. Greenberg said. "They could have got a toxic dose of some drug by accident. In the oatmeal, most likely. I couldn't help thinking that the oatmeal was relevant to our problem. At any rate, the drug idea was very persuasive."

"So was Greenberg," Dr. Pellitteri remarked with a smile. "Actually, it was the only explanation in sight that seemed to account for everything we knew about the clinical and environmental picture."

"All we had to do now was prove it," Dr. Greenberg went on mildly. "I asked Pellitteri to get a blood sample from each of the men before leaving the hospital for a look at the cafeteria. We agreed he would send the specimens to the city toxicologist, Dr. Alexander O. Gettler, for an overnight analysis. I wanted to know if the blood contained methemoglobin. Methemoglobin is a compound that's formed only when any one of several drugs enters the blood. Gettler's report would tell us if we were at least on the right track. That is, it would give us a yes-or-no answer on drugs. If the answer was yes, then we could go on from there to identify the particular drug. How we would go about that would depend on what Pellitteri was able to turn up at the cafeteria. In the meantime, there was nothing for me to do but wait for their reports. I'd theorized myself hoarse."

Dr. Pellitteri, having attended to his bloodletting with reasonable dispatch, reached the Eclipse Cafeteria at around five o'clock. "It was about what I'd expected," he told me. "Strictly a horse market, and dirtier than most. The sort of place where you can get a full meal for fifteen cents. There was a grind house on one side, a cigar store on the other, and the 'L' overhead. Incidentally, the Eclipse went out of business a year or so after I was there, but that had nothing to do with us. It was just a coincidence. Well, the place looked deserted and the door was locked. I knocked, and a man came out of the back and let me in. He was one of our people, a health inspector for the Bureau of Food and Drugs, named Weinberg. His bureau had stepped into the case as a matter of routine, because of the reference to a restaurant in the notification report. I was glad to see him and to have his help. For one thing, he had put a temporary embargo on everything in the cafeteria. That's why it was closed up. His main job, though, was to check the place for violations of the sanitation code. He was finding plenty."

"Let me read you a few of Weinberg's findings," Dr. Greenberg said, extracting a paper from the folder on his desk. "None of them had any direct bearing on our problem, but I think they'll give you a good idea of what the Eclipse was like — what too many restaurants are like. This copy of his report lists fifteen specific violations. Here they are: 'Premises heavily infested with roaches. Fly infestation throughout premises. Floor defective in rear part of dining room. Kitchen walls and ceiling encrusted with grease and soot. Kitchen floor encrusted with dirt. Refuse under kitchen fixtures. Sterilizing facilities inadequate. Sink defective. Floor and walls at serving tables and coffee urns encrusted with dirt. Kitchen utensils encrusted with dirt and grease. Storage-cellar walls, ceiling, and floor encrusted with dirt. Floor and shelves in cellar covered with refuse and useless material. Cellar ceiling defective. Sewer pipe leaking. Open sewer line in cellar.' Well . . ." He gave me a squeamish smile and stuck the paper back in the folder.

"I can see it now," Dr. Pellitteri said. "And smell it. Especially the kitchen, where I spent most of my time. Weinberg had the proprietor and the cook out there, and I talked to them while he prowled around. They were very coöperative. Naturally. They were scared to death. They knew nothing about gas in the place and there was no sign of any, so I went to work on the food. None of what had been prepared for breakfast that morning was left. That, of course, would have been too much to hope for. But I was able to get together some of the kind of stuff that had gone into the men's breakfast, so that we could make a chemical determination at the Department. What I took was ground coffee, sugar, a mixture of evaporated milk and water that passed for cream, some bakery rolls, a five-pound carton of dry oatmeal, and some salt. The salt had been used in preparing the oatmeal. That morning, like every morning, the cook told me, he had prepared six gallons of oatmeal, enough to serve around a hundred and twenty-five people. To make it, he used five pounds of dry cereal, four gallons of water — regular city water — and a handful of salt. That was his term — a handful. There was an open gallon can of salt standing on the stove. He said the handful he'd put in that morning's oatmeal had come from that. He refilled the can on the stove every morning from a big supply can. He pointed out the big can — it was up on a shelf — and as I was getting it down to take with me, I saw another can, just like it, nearby. I took that one down, too. It was also full of salt, or, rather, something that looked like salt. The proprietor said it wasn't salt. He said it was saltpetre — sodium nitrate — that he used in corning beef and in making pastrami. Well, there isn't any harm in saltpetre; it doesn't even act as an anti-aphrodisiac, as a lot of people seem to think. But I wrapped it up with the other loot and took it along, just for fun. The fact is, I guess, everything in that damn place looked like poison."

After Dr. Pellitteri had deposited his loot with a Health Department chemist, Andrew J. Pensa, who promised to have a report ready by the following afternoon, he dined hurriedly at a restaurant in which he had confidence and returned to Chatham Square. There he spent the evening making the rounds of the lodging houses in the neighborhood. He had heard at Mr. Pensa's office that an eleventh blue man had been admitted to the hospital, and before going home he wanted to make sure that no other victims had been overlooked. By midnight, having covered all the likely places and having rechecked the downtown hospitals, he was satisfied. He repaired to his office and composed a formal progress report for Dr. Greenberg. Then he went home and to bed.

The next morning, Tuesday, Dr. Pellitteri dropped by the Eclipse, which was still closed but whose proprietor and staff he had told to return for questioning. Dr. Pellitteri had another talk with the proprietor and the cook. He also had a few inconclusive words with the rest of the cafeteria's employees — two dishwashers, a busboy, and a counterman. As he was leaving, the cook, who had apparently passed an uneasy night with his conscience, remarked that it was possible that he had absent-mindedly refilled the salt can on the stove from the one that contained saltpetre. "That was interesting," Dr. Pellitteri told me, "even though such a possibility had already occurred to me, and even though I didn't know whether it was important or not. I assured him that he had nothing to worry about. We had been certain all along that nobody had deliberately poisoned the old men." From the Eclipse, Dr. Pellitteri went on to Dr. Greenberg's office, where Dr. Gettler's report was waiting.

"Gettler's test for methemoglobin was positive," Dr. Greenberg said. "It had to be a drug now. Well, so far so good. Then we heard from Pensa."

"Greenberg almost fell out of his chair when he read Pensa's report," Dr. Pellitteri observed cheerfully.

"That's an exaggeration," Dr. Greenberg said. "I'm not easily dumfounded. We're inured to the incredible around here. Why, a few years ago we had a case involving some numskull who stuck a fistful of potassium-thiocyanate crystals, a very nasty poison, in the coils of an office water cooler, just for a practical joke. However, I can't deny that Pensa rather taxed our credulity. What he had found was that the small salt can and the one that was supposed to be full of sodium nitrate both contained sodium *nitrite*. The other food samples, incidentally, were O.K."

"That also taxed my credulity," Dr. Pellitteri said.

Dr. Greenberg smiled. "There's a great deal of difference between nitrate and nitrite," he continued. "Their only similarity, which is an unfortunate one, is that they both look and taste more or less like ordinary table salt. Sodium nitrite isn't the most powerful poison in the world, but a little of it will do a lot of harm. If you remember, I said before that this case was almost without precedent — only ten outbreaks like it on record. Ten is practically none. In fact, sodium-nitrite poisoning is so unusual that some of the standard texts on toxicology don't even mention it. So Pensa's report was pretty startling. But we accepted it, of course, without question or hesitation. Facts are facts. And we were glad to. It seemed to explain everything very nicely. What I've been saying about sodium-nitrite poisoning doesn't mean that sodium nitrite itself is rare. Actually, it's fairly common. It's used in the manufacture of dyes and as a medical drug. We use it in treating certain heart conditions and for high blood pressure. But it also has another important use, one that made its presence at the Eclipse sound plausible. In recent years, and particularly during the war, sodium nitrite has been used as a substitute for sodium nitrate in preserving meat. The government permits it but stipulates that the finished meat must not contain more than one part of sodium nitrite per five thousand parts of meat. Cooking will safely destroy enough of that small quantity of the drug." Dr. Greenberg shrugged. "Well, Pellitteri had had the cook pick up a handful of salt — the same amount, as nearly as possible, as went into the oatmeal — and then had taken this to his office and found that it weighed approximately a hundred grams. So we didn't have to think twice to realize that the proportion of nitrite in that batch of cereal was considerably higher than one to five thousand. Roughly, it must have been around one to about eighty before cooking destroyed part of the nitrite. It certainly looked as though Gettler, Pensa, and the cafeteria cook between them had given us our answer. I called up Gettler and told him what Pensa had discovered and asked him to run a specific test for nitrites on his blood samples. He had, as a matter of course, held some blood back for later examination. His confirmation came through in a couple of hours. I went home that night feeling pretty good."

Dr. Greenberg's serenity was a fugitive one. He awoke on Wednesday morning troubled in mind. A question had occurred to him that he was unable to ignore. "Something like a hundred and twenty-five people ate oatmeal at the Eclipse that morning," he said to me, "but only eleven of them got sick. Why? The undeniable fact that those eleven old men were made sick by the ingestion of a toxic dose of sodium nitrite wasn't enough to rest on. I wanted to know exactly how much sodium nitrite each portion of that cooked oatmeal had contained. With Pensa's help again, I found out. We prepared a batch just like the one the cook had made on Monday. Then Pensa measured out six ounces, the size of the average portion served at the Eclipse, and analyzed it. It contained two and a half grains of sodium nitrite. That explained why the hundred and fourteen other people did not become ill. The toxic dose of sodium nitrite is three grains. But it didn't explain how each of our eleven old men had received an additional half grain. It seemed extremely unlikely that the extra touch of nitrite had been in the oatmeal when it was served. It had to come in later. Then I began to get a glimmer. Some people sprinkle a little salt, instead of sugar, on hot cereal. Suppose, I thought, that the busboy, or whoever had the job of keeping the table salt shakers filled, had made the same mistake that the cook had. It seemed plausible. Pellitteri was out of the office — I've forgotten where — so I got Food and Drugs to step over to the Eclipse, which was still under embargo, and bring back the shakers for Pensa to work on. There were seventeen of them, all good-sized, one for each table. Sixteen contained either pure sodium chloride or just a few inconsequential traces of sodium nitrite mixed in with the real salt, but the other was point thirty-seven per cent nitrite. That one was enough. A spoonful of that salt contained a bit more than half a grain."

"I went over to the hospital Thursday morning," Dr. Pellitteri said. "Greenberg wanted me to check the table-salt angle with the men. They could tie the case up neatly for us. I drew a blank. They'd been discharged the night before, and God only knew where they were."

"Naturally," Dr. Greenberg said, "it would have been nice to know for a fact that the old boys all sat at a certain table and that all of them put about a spoonful of salt from that particular shaker on their oatmeal, but it wasn't essential. I was morally certain that they had. There just wasn't any other explanation. There was one other question, however. Why did they use so *much* salt? For my own peace of mind, I wanted to know. All of a sudden, I remembered Pellitteri had said they were all heavy drinkers. Well, several recent clinical studies have demonstrated that there is usually a subnormal concentration of sodium chloride in the blood of alcoholics. Either they don't eat enough to get sufficient salt or they lose it more rapidly than other people do, or both. Whatever the reasons are, the conclusion was all I needed. Any animal, you know, whether a mouse or a man, tends to try to obtain a necessary substance that his body lacks. The final question had been answered."

A Man from Mexico

SMALLPOX is an ancient and immoderately ferocious disease of Oriental origin that shares with plague, cholera, and epidemic typhus the distinction of having once or twice in the past five hundred years come fairly close to eradicating the human race. It is less unmanageable now. A full-fledged smallpox epidemic has been nearly unheard of since the late nineteenth century. Except in a few parts of the world — most of them easygoing — the appearance of even a handful of cases is an unusual occurrence. The only countries in which serious outbreaks have been at all frequent in recent years are India, Japan, Siam, Korea, British East Africa, Venezuela, and the United States.

About the best that can be said for smallpox is that it is somewhat less barbaric than plague. Plague is almost invariably fatal. Smallpox strikes with varying degrees of intensity and in some epidemics there have been so many mild cases that a large majority of the victims have recovered, but the disease is by no means always so benign. At its worst — when it is known as black, or hemorrhagic, smallpox — it is almost always lethal. Victims of even the blandest attacks of smallpox occasionally succumb to one or another of several complications to which the disease is hospitable, among them septic poisoning and broncho-pneumonia, and those fortunate enough to survive an attack are often crippled for life. Blindness is a possible, though uncommon, consequence. Few have ever emerged scot-free from an attack of smallpox. Because of the pustular eruptions which characterize the disease, and from which its name is derived, it is almost certain to be permanently disfiguring. It can also be one of the most unnerving and repulsive of ailments. "The patient often becomes a dripping, unrecognizable mass of pus by the seventh or eighth day of eruption," Dr. Archibald L. Hoyne, medical superintendent of the Chicago Municipal Contagious Disease Hospital, has noted in a clinical study. "The putrid odor is stifling, the temperature often high [107° has been authoritatively reported], and the patient frequently in a wild state of delirium." Moreover, unlike plague, cholera, typhus, and many other deadly infections, the transmission of which is usually limited to either a carrier insect or contaminated drinking water, smallpox is abundantly contagious. Some epidemiologists consider it the most contagious of all diseases, including measles and the common cold.

The cause of smallpox is a durable virus. It enters the body through the respiratory system and is present in the exhalations of its victims for hours, and very likely days, before the apparent onset of illness. It is prolifically communicable during the entire course of the disease and may even be contracted from a victim some hours after his death. It can be conveyed by clothing, books, or letters, and there is good reason to believe that it is as readily airborne as dust. Nobody is naturally immune to smallpox, survival of one attack is no absolute assurance of future immunity, and, since both nonagenarians and unborn babies have been stricken, susceptibility is seemingly unrelated to age. A specific cure has yet to be discovered, and medical treatment, while desirable, is merely palliative. However, smallpox is not unavoidable. It is, in fact, among the few diseases against which certain immunization is possible. "There is no more certain truth in all the world," Dr. Hoyne has written, "than that an individual properly vaccinated with potent lymph [living virus] cannot contract smallpox in any manner whatsoever."

Many physicians are inclined these days to regard smallpox as an anachronism. This assumption, though infirm, is by no means unreasonable. The development of a reliable method of preventing the disease is not only one of scientific medicine's loftiest triumphs but one of its earliest; by illuminating the mechanics of disease in general, vaccination, which dates from the eighteenth century, inspired the immunological discoveries of Pasteur, von Behring, Ehrlich, and others. Long before the discovery of vaccination, it was possible to exert some preventive control over smallpox. In the third century before Christ, pioneering healers in India became aware that the injection of a minute quantity of virulent smallpox matter into a healthy person often produced a painless seizure and subsequent immunity. Inoculation, as this procedure came to be known, was introduced into Europe, by way of Turkey, in 1717, or thereabouts, and was widely practiced on the Continent and elsewhere until vaccination turned up, a couple of generations later. The first deliberate vaccination was performed by an English dairy farmer named Benjamin Jesty in 1774. Jesty had observed that milkmaids who had suffered an attack of vaccinia, or cowpox — a harmless occupational malaise of bovine derivation — seemed to be impervious to smallpox. He conceived the useful notion of relating that barnyard phenomenon to the technique of inoculation, and, using lymph from an ailing cow, immunized himself and his wife and children, at least to his own satisfaction. As a vaccinator, Jesty apparently confined his efforts to the family circle. It is possible that Dr. Edward Jenner, a British physician who is more commonly celebrated as the discoverer of vaccination, never heard of him. Dr. Jenner vaccinated his first patient in 1796, with the same sort of lymph Jesty had employed. Two years later, he published his revolutionary treatise "An Inquiry into the Causes and Effects of the Variolæ Vaccinæ, a Disease Discovered in Some of the Western Counties of England, Particularly Gloucestershire, and Known by the Name of the Cowpox." Inoculation has two drawbacks as a smallpox preventive. In addition to being uncomfortably speculative, the seizure it brings on is as contagious as the real thing. Since the virus of cowpox, though the disease is probably a form of smallpox, is consistently effective but innocuous, vaccination has neither of these imperfections. Its only flaw, an easily remedied one, is that the immunity conferred by it diminishes with the passage of time.

The model efficiency of vaccination was almost at once recognized throughout the world. The first American vaccinator, Dr. Benjamin Waterhouse, professor of physics at the Harvard University Medical School, immunized his first patient in 1800. Not long after, in England, the Bishop of Worcester set a clerical precedent by commending the practice to his communicants. In 1805, Napoleon made vaccination compulsory in the French Army, a precaution that has since been taken by the military authorities of nearly all nations, and persuasively urged it upon civilians, not only in France but in Italy as well. Compulsory vaccination of everybody was presently instituted in many countries—

Bavaria (1807), Norway, Denmark, and Iceland (1810), Sweden (1814), the German states (1818), Great Britain (1853), Rumania (1874), Hungary (1876), and Austria (1886). Other countries have since become equally thorough, but the United States is not among them. Compulsory vaccination has always been considered unnecessary here, except for the armed forces. In some states and in some cities (New York City is one), it is required only as a prerequisite to attending elementary school. Even this gentle bit of coercion has occasionally been opposed by patriots as tyrannical.

In spite of this country's somewhat indulgent attitude toward smallpox prevention, the disease is no longer, at least statistically, a very active menace here. A visitation in 1901–02 that centered upon New York City and caused seven hundred and twenty deaths in this area is usually cited as the last high-velocity epidemic. However, smallpox still turns up; generally, more than a hundred cases of it occur in the United States every year, and in one recent year, 1930, nearly forty-nine thousand were reported — an incidence, considering the ease with which the disease can be prevented, of almost astronomical proportions. Ordinarily, the cases are widely scattered, but there have been numerous concentrated outbreaks even since the First World War. A hundred and sixty people died in one, in 1921, in Kansas City. Another, later that year, in Denver, caused thirty-seven deaths. In 1924, in Detroit, out of sixteen hundred and ten cases a hundred and sixty-three were fatal. There were twenty deaths during an outbreak in the Puget Sound area around Seattle in 1945. In the spring of 1947, to the unnatural astonishment of the press, the public, and most physicians, smallpox reappeared, after an absence of not quite eight years, in New York City. It struck, altogether, twelve men, women, and children. Two of them died. Largely because of dazzling good luck and the dispatch with which the Department of Health tracked down and sequestered several hundred people presumed to have been exposed to the disease, the outbreak proved to be one of the mildest on record. It could have been hair-raising. Dr. Morris Greenberg, director of the Department's Bureau of Preventable Diseases, has estimated that at the time the first victim died, only about two million of the city's nearly eight million inhabitants had any degree of immunity whatever to smallpox.

The New York City Health Department, to which the appearance of a serious communicable disease anywhere in the city must be promptly reported, learned of the 1947 outbreak toward noon on Friday, March 28th. Its informant was Dr. Dorothea M. Tolle, medical superintendent of Willard Parker Hospital, a municipal institution for the treatment of contagious diseases, at the foot of East Fifteenth Street. Her report, which she made by telephone, as is customary when a potentially fast-moving contagion is involved, was inconclusive but disheartening. Two patients, whose trouble was at first believed to be chicken pox, had overnight developed eruptions that looked alarmingly like those of smallpox. Dr. Edward M. Bernecker, Commissioner of Hospitals, and Dr. Ralph S. Muckenfuss, director of the Bureau of Laboratories, had both been apprised of the occurrence, she added, and the latter was arranging for a definitive laboratory analysis of material taken from the patients. Dr. Tolle's lack of certainty, which was shared by her deputy, Dr. Irving Klein, and the other members of the Willard Parker staff, was not surprising. Smallpox has always been an elusive disease to diagnose in its early stages, the symptoms that mark its onset — chills, fever, headache, and nausea — being indistinguishable from those of influenza, malaria, and typhoid fever. Bedside recognition of it at any stage is difficult now, for contemporary physicians generally find even the rash peculiar to the disease — a rash that emerges on the third or fourth day of illness and becomes pustular by the eighth — more confusing than enlightening. One reason for this diagnostic stumbling is that many doctors currently in practice have never seen a case of smallpox. Another is that several other rashy disorders — among them chicken pox, measles, scarlet fever, scabies, acne, impetigo, syphilis, and ulcerative endocarditis — are more insistently prevalent and, consequently, come more readily to mind. The thought of smallpox forced itself upon Dr. Tolle and Dr. Klein that Friday morning in 1947 mainly because the rash displayed by the two invalids was, providentially, of an almost classic clarity.

By one o'clock, copies of Dr. Tolle's report had been distributed to all administrative officers of the Department and an investigation of the cases was briskly under way. Its pattern, despite the unusual nature of the alarm, was routine and confidential. As a preliminary defensive measure, Dr. Bernecker and Dr. Israel Weinstein, then Commissioner of Health, ordered a speedy vaccination of everybody at Willard Parker — doctors, nurses, lay employees, and patients — and instructed the authorities there not to admit any visitor who declined to be vaccinated on the spot. A summary clinical inquiry was at the same time, and as a matter of course, undertaken by Dr. David A. Singer, chief diagnostician of the Manhattan division of the Bureau of Preventable Diseases. He lit out for the hospital the moment the notification reached him. He found both suspected victims flushed, feverish, freshly vaccinated, and tucked away in individual, glassed-in cubicles in a remote corner of an isolation building. One of them was a twenty-six-year-old Puerto Rican, who, because of the turn events took in his instance, can be specifically identified as Ismael Acosta. The other was a Negro infant, Patricia G——, aged twenty-two months, whose name, like the names of most patients under such circumstances, can be given only in part. Dr. Singer's diagnosis, which he presently telephoned to Dr. Greenberg, his superior, tentatively confirmed the suspicions of Dr. Tolle and Dr. Klein. Dr. Muckenfuss, meanwhile, within an hour after being alerted by Dr. Tolle, had obtained some fluid from the lesions of the two patients and dispatched the samples by plane to Dr. Joseph Smadel, director of the United States Army Medical School Laboratory, in Washington, for full-scale examination. His choice of the Army Laboratory was instinctive; at the time it was the closest to New York of the few laboratories in the country that were equipped to perform the intricate and time-consuming tests by which the presence of smallpox virus can be detected. Then, before turning his attention to other things, Dr. Muckenfuss got in touch with Dr. Weinstein. He told him that a dependable yes-or-no answer from Dr. Smadel should be along in about a week.

The cheerless uniformity of the clinical opinions of Dr. Tolle, Dr. Klein, and Dr. Singer gave Dr. Weinstein little reason to hope for a relaxing word from Dr. Smadel, but he felt restrained by the lack of absolute certainty from authorizing at the moment a far-reaching investigation. He preferred, so long as there was any doubt, to shield the city from the shrieks and speculations of the press. His discretion did not, however, encourage departmental idleness. The next morning, Saturday, March 29th, as part of the undercover investigation, a couple of the most inquisitive operatives in the Bureau of Preventable Diseases were quietly assigned to assist Dr. Singer. Their job was to discover where and how, if Acosta and Patricia did have smallpox, the disease had been contracted. To this end, with the lively coöperation of Dr. Tolle and Dr. Klein, they fixed their attention on the hospital records. Taken together, the dossiers of the two patients made provocative reading. Acosta was married lived in the East Bronx, was employed as a porter at Bellevu Hospital, and had reached Willard Parker on Thursday, March 27th, having first spent two days in the dermatologic ward at Bellevue. The baby had been admitted to Willard Parker six days before Acosta. She had fallen sick on March 19th. Two days later, her parents had taken her to a clinic near their home, in Harlem, and from there she had been sent at once to Willard Parker. What quickened the interest of the investigators was that neither of the patients was a newcomer to the hospital. Both had been there previously, and at the same time. Less than a month before, Acosta had spent a couple of weeks — from February 27th to March 11th — at Willard Parker, with the mumps. Patricia's earlier visit, the outcome of an attack of croup, had lasted from February 28th to March 13th. Dr. Singer and his colleagues, mindful that the incubation period of smallpox is generally around twelve to fourteen days and never more than twenty-one, made themselves comfortable and began to absorb this instructive set of coincidences. By Saturday evening, they had been led to the somewhat reassuring suspicion that Acosta and Patricia had acquired the disease from the same source. Over the weekend, a third and equally probable case of smallpox was uncovered in Willard Parker. The new victim was a boy of two and a half, named John F——, who had been in the hospital, suffering from whooping cough, since March 6th. The fact that his had been an uninterrupted confinement strengthened the investigators' hunch to a near certainty. They concluded that Acosta, Patricia, and John had contracted smallpox at the hospital, from somebody who had been there between March 6th and March 13th.

The unflattering implications of this conclusion embarrassed Dr. Tolle and Dr. Klein, but only momentarily. They calmed themselves with the reflection that diagnostic infallibility is more often the aspiration than the achievement of any hospital staff. To Dr. Klein, the experience was even salutary, and he emerged from it both unruffled and inspired. Memory revived in him with the abruptness of revelation. Early in March, he now recalled, there had been a patient at Willard Parker in whom one physician had fleetingly thought he detected indications of smallpox. Dr. Klein guided the investigators back to the files and, after some digging, produced the record of the patient he had in mind. It was that of a man named Eugene La Bar, and the case it described was morbid, chaotic, and dismaying. La Bar, an American, had lived since 1940 in Mexico City, where he had desultorily engaged in exporting leather goods. He was forty-seven years old, married, and childless. Toward the end of February, he and his wife had left Mexico City and headed for New York, travelling by bus. It was their intention to go right on to Readfield, Maine, to view a farm that Mrs. La Bar had just inherited near there, but La Bar became ill during the journey. His discomfort, which he attempted to relieve by frequent doses of aspirin, codeine, Nembutal, and phenobarbital, consisted of a headache and a severe pain in the back of the neck. By the time the couple reached New York, La Bar felt too unwell to go any farther.

As far as could be ascertained from the record, he had gone at once to the clinic at Bellevue, where an examining physician, observing that he had a fever of 105° and an odd rash on his face and hands, admitted him to the hospital's dermatologic ward. The date of his admittance was March 5th, a Wednesday. Three days later, on March 8th, La Bar was transferred to Willard Parker, his condition having baffled and finally frightened the Bellevue dermatologists. He arrived there more dead than alive. The rash by then covered his entire body, and it was pustular and hemorrhagic. It was this rash that prompted one of the Willard Parker doctors to offer a halfhearted diagnosis of smallpox. It also impelled him to vaccinate Mrs. La Bar when she called at the hospital that afternoon to inquire about her husband. Then the physician dropped the theory. His reasons were plausible. A freehand analysis of material taken from the lesions did not appear to support his guess; the rash, upon closer scrutiny, was not strikingly typical of smallpox; La Bar had an old but well-developed vaccination scar; and Mrs. La Bar insisted that her husband could not possibly have been in recent contact with anybody suffering from the disease. Three other diagnoses that had also been more or less seriously considered were enumerated in the record. One, suggested by the vigor and variety of the painkillers with which La Bar had stuffed himself, was drug poisoning. Another was Kaposi's varicelliform eruption, a kind of edema complicated by pustules. The third was erythema multiforme, an acute skin infection, and this had seemed the likeliest. La Bar lay in an agony of delirium for two days. On Monday morning, March 10th, his fever suddenly vanished and he felt almost well. Late that afternoon, he died. An autopsy disclosed, among other internal dishevelments, an enlarged spleen, a friable liver, and multiple hemorrhages in the viscera and the lungs. The final entry on the record was the cause of death: "Erythema multiforme, with laryngo-tracheo-bronchitis and bronchopneumonia." It was not a deduction in which Dr. Klein and the Health Department physicians, whose wits had been sharpened by hindsight, were tempted to concur. Their persuasion was that they had just read a forceful account of an unusually virulent attack of black smallpox.

On the morning of Friday, April 4th, the report from Dr. Smadel came through. It was affirmative; both Acosta and Patricia had smallpox. (Subsequently, Dr. Smadel was able to say the same of John and several others, including the deceased La Bar; some material taken from the latter's lesions for the test made at the hospital had, it developed, fortunately been preserved.) Dr. Weinstein received the report without marked consternation. His reaction was almost one of relief. It delivered him from the misery of retaining an increasingly unreasonable doubt. It also propelled him into rapid motion. He notified the United States Public Health Service of the outbreak. Then he had a word of counsel with Dr. Bernecker. After that, he assembled the administrative officers of the Departments of Health and of Hospitals for a briefing on tactics. Next, waving Dr. Greenberg's agents out into the open, he set a full-dress investigation in motion. At two o'clock Dr. Weinstein broke the news to the press at a conference in his office. His statement included an exhortation. "It is not surprising that smallpox has reappeared in this city," he said. "The Health Department has stated many times that we are exposed to communicable diseases occurring in this and neighboring countries. The danger of a widespread epidemic is slight, because our population is for the most part protected by vaccination. Smallpox is one of the most communicable of all diseases, and the only known preventive measure is vaccination. Anyone in the city who has never been vaccinated, or who has not been vaccinated since early childhood, should get this protection at once. Smallpox is a serious disease that may cause permanent disfigurement, damage to vital organs, and even death. With vaccination, a simple and harmless procedure, available to all, there is absolutely no excuse for anyone to remain unprotected." Dr. Weinstein was aware, as he spoke, that his advice was somewhat sounder than his optimism.

The public investigation, like the plainclothes reconnaissance that had preceded it, was accompanied by a quarantine measure; the dermatologic ward at Bellevue was closed to visitors who could not give convincing assurance that they had recently been vaccinated. In addition, vaccination of the entire population of the hospital commenced — a considerable task in itself, which was entrusted to the Department of Hospitals and the Bellevue staff. The rest of the undertaking was handled, without complaint, by the Bureau of Preventable Diseases. It involved the tracking down, the vaccination, and the continued surveillance during the smallpox period of incubation of every person who was known to have been exposed to the disease. Dr. Greenberg's medical staff consists of, in addition to himself and Dr. Singer, three full-time inspectors and thirty-five part-time men. He put them all to work on the task. By nightfall on Friday, less than twelve hours after the arrival of Dr. Smadel's report, Dr. Greenberg's men had called upon, examined, and vaccinated some two hundred potential victims and were on the trail of several hundred others. These two groups comprised all the residents of the apartment buildings in which the Acostas and Patricia's family lived, everyone who had been in the Harlem clinic on the day of Patricia's visit, and everyone who had set foot in Willard Parker between March 8th and March 27th or in the Bellevue dermatologic ward between March 5th and March 8th or between March 25th and March 27th, but they did not comprise all those who might conceivably have been infected. This was no reflection on the resourcefulness of the Bureau men. Dr. Weinstein and his associates had known from the outset that the city contained innumerable possible smallpox cases who were beyond the timely reach of any investigators. They were the people among whom La Bar, on March 5th, and Patricia, on March 21st, and Acosta, on March 25th, had passed on their way to the hospital. It was largely Acosta's means of getting there that prompted Dr. Weinstein to try to stimulate in the public an orderly but general desire for vaccination. La Bar had travelled in the moderate seclusion of a cab, and Patricia had left the clinic in an ambulance. Acosta had taken the subway and a crosstown bus.

The immediate response to Dr. Weinstein's exhortation, which he quickly condensed for press and radio use into the slogan "Be Sure, Be Safe, Get Vaccinated!," was only mildly gratifying. Undismayed, he instructed the Bureau of Laboratories to at once set about converting its bulk supplies of vaccine into handy, one-dose units and to make these available without charge, through drugstores, to all physicians and, directly, to all hospitals and to the city's twenty-one district health centers. He issued a public statement emphasizing that the protection he recommended was free as well as simple and harmless. Over the weekend, his meaning appeared to have been caught only by the prudent and the panicky, but on Monday, April 7th, an encouragingly widened comprehension was perceptible. There was good reason. Two new cases of suspected smallpox had turned up and been proclaimed. Acosta's wife, who was twenty-six years old and in the seventh month of pregnancy, was one of them. She had become ill at her home on Saturday night. The following morning the inspector assigned to patrol the building took one alert look at her and summoned a Willard Parker ambulance. The other was a Cuban, who, as it later turned out, had nothing worse than chicken pox, but by the time his case was correctly diagnosed, another case of smallpox had come to light. This was on Thursday, April 10th. The patient was a forty-three-year-old wanderer named Herman G——, whose condition had come to the attention of a physician in the dermatologic ward at Bellevue, where he had been confined for treatment of syphilis since March 10th. The next day, April 11th, still another victim was reported. He was a businessman of fifty-seven named Harry T——, and his case, too, was discovered in the Bellevue dermatologic ward. He had been admitted there, suffering from lymphoblastoma, on March 19th. His misfortune, as the newspapers loudly and uneasily pointed out, brought the number of smallpox cases to seven. It also had the effect of abruptly increasing to around a hundred thousand the number of people who had heeded Dr. Weinstein's admonition.

While dutifully notifying the United States Public Health Service of the outbreak and its transcontinental origin, Dr. Weinstein had expressed a normal interest in Mrs. La Bar's whereabouts and the state of her health. It was his understanding, he said, that she had continued on to Maine soon after her husband's funeral; nothing had been heard from her since, although the true cause of her husband's death had been widely publicized. As might be expected, Dr. Weinstein's curiosity concerning Mrs. La Bar was at least equalled by that of the Public Health Service. He was promised an early reply, and on Wednesday, April 9th, his day was enlivened by a report from the Service on its findings. They were numerous and in some respects reassuring, in others highly disturbing. Mrs. La Bar was at the home of a relative in East Winthrop, Maine, and in excellent health. Information obtained from her had enabled the Service to alert the health authorities in the towns at which the La Bars' bus had stopped — Laredo, San Antonio, Dallas, Tulsa, Joplin, St. Louis, Indianapolis, Cincinnati, and Pittsburgh. None had reported any local evidence of smallpox. La Bar's illness apparently hadn't reached a highly contagious stage during the journey. What distressed Dr. Weinstein was the disclosure that the La Bars had arrived in New York from Mexico City on Saturday afternoon, March 1st. This meant that they had been in the city five days before La Bar finally tottered into Bellevue. During that time, they had stayed at a hotel, which the Health Department has charitably never seen fit to identify. Fortunately, because of La Bar's unrelenting aches and pains, they seldom left their room. The only time they went outside the hotel, as far as Mrs. La Bar could recall, was on the Monday after their arrival here, when they took a stroll up Fifth Avenue and made a few trivial purchases at McCreery's, at a ten-cent store, and at the Knox hat shop. The report added that Mrs. La Bar's earlier reticence had been caused by a lifelong aversion to red tape.

A somewhat similar reticence was discovered in an assistant manager of the La Bars' hotel by a squad of Dr. Greenberg's agents who stopped by later that Wednesday. It was their intention to vaccinate all the hotel's employees and permanent residents and to gather the names and addresses of all transient guests registered there between March 1st and March 5th. The opposition that they encountered was rigid, but it was not prolonged. It vanished at a thawing murmur from Dr. Greenberg over the telephone to the effect that the full text of Mrs. La Bar's memoir could easily be substituted for the tactfully expurgated version, omitting the name of the hotel, that was then being prepared for the press. His words induced a cordiality of such intensity that the manager himself trotted out the records and asked to be the first to bare his arm. By bedtime Wednesday night, the inspectors had made a satisfying start on both their tasks, and they finished up the following day. Approximately three thousand people had spent one or more of the first five days of March under the same roof as La Bar. Nearly all were from out of town, and the names and addresses of these, who included residents of twenty-nine states, were transmitted to the health authorities of those states. Dr. Greenberg's men added what guests there had been from New York City to their already generous list of local suspects. In time, all the three thousand, except for a few dozen adventurers who had registered under spurious names, were hunted down and, as it happily turned out, given a clean bill of health.

Meanwhile, Dr. Weinstein and Dr. Greenberg had decided that there wasn't much they could do in the way of disinfecting the La Bars' month-old trail up Fifth Avenue. They tried to console themselves with the realization that private physicians and the district health centers were experiencing another substantial increase in the demand for safety and certainty. This followed the newspaper publication, on Thursday, of Mrs. La Bar's censored revelations, which contained a discomfortingly vague reference to "a midtown hotel," in and about which La Bar had passed five days at nearly the peak of his contagiousness. Practically all the hotels in Manhattan at which a transient would be likely to stop are in the midtown area.

Bright and early Saturday morning, April 12th, there was more unpleasant news. It was relayed to Dr. Weinstein by the New York State Department of Health, and it came from the village of Millbrook, in Dutchess County. A boy of four, Vernon L——, whose family lived in the Bronx, had been sick there for several days with what Dr. Smadel, in whom the state health authorities also had confidence, had just diagnosed as smallpox. The boy, an inmate of the Cardinal Hayes Convalescent Home, on the outskirts of town, was not, it appeared, critically ill. The source of the infection was no mystery. Before being admitted to the Home, on March 13th, Vernon had spent eighteen days, from February 21st to March 10th, at Willard Parker, under treatment for scarlet fever. He was one of a number of Willard Parker alumni no longer in the city whom the state investigators had been asked to trace. The news of the Millbrook case was conveyed to Dr. Weinstein by telephone. The morning brought him two more agitating calls. One was from Dr. Muckenfuss and the other from Dr. Tolle. Dr. Muckenfuss reported that the municipal supply of vaccine was going fast. Two hundred thousand units had been distributed during the past week, and no more than that number were still on hand. Dr. Tolle called to say that Mrs. Acosta had just died.

At one-thirty that afternoon, Dr. Weinstein, accompanied

by Dr. Bernecker and a couple of his other associates, hopped around to Gracie Mansion for a candid chat with Mayor O'Dwyer, whom they found enduring an instant of repose. It had been Dr. Weinstein's original and commendable determination to spare the Mayor any direct concern with the calamity. Dr. Muckenfuss's information, on top of everything else, had compelled him to change his mind. After Dr. Weinstein and his colleagues had successfully communicated their uneasiness to the Mayor, they divulged a more specific reason for their visit. They asked for an appropriation of five hundred thousand dollars. Most of this sum, which, after a little ritualistic sparring, the Mayor agreed to wheedle out of the Board of Estimate, would be expended for vaccine, Dr. Weinstein explained, and the rest for other extraordinary expenses of the Health and Hospital Departments, including the hiring of a thousand doctors and a couple of hundred clerks to man additional public vaccination centers in various parts of the city. Then, also at the request of Dr. Weinstein, the Mayor led the group down to City Hall, where at five o'clock he met in his office with the commissioners of all municipal departments and instructed them to see to it that no city employee delayed an instant in getting vaccinated. Before knocking off for the day, the Mayor called in the press, invited the photographers to unlimber their cameras, and allowed Dr. Weinstein to vaccinate him. This, he pointed out, was his fifth vaccination in six years, the others having been acquired during his service in the Army, but it was better to be safe than sorry.

Over the weekend, the words and insinuating example of Mayor O'Dwyer, which were supplemented, on the air at nine o'clock Sunday evening, by a sudden, inflammatory chirp from Walter Winchell, resulted in a powerful quickening of the instinct for self-preservation, and this was still further heightened by word from the convalescent home in Millbrook that three more smallpox cases — two of them child inmates and the other an elderly nun on the staff of the institution — had been discovered there. Eighty-four thousand people, including hundreds in the remotest wastes of Staten Island, were vaccinated on Monday. On Tuesday, following the announcement of yet another case of smallpox originating at Bellevue — that of a sixty-year-old man who had been in the hospital suffering from a serious skin ailment for many months — two hundred thousand more were vaccinated. So great was the drain on the municipal reserves of vaccine that the Mayor summoned before him representatives of all the big pharmaceutical firms that have plants or offices here and extracted from them a collective promise to make available to the city an abundant and immediate supply of the preparation. Pending the fulfillment of their pledge, he arranged, over the telephone, for an interim loan of vaccine from the Army and Navy. Wednesday night, in the course of announcing that emergency clinics would be opened the following morning in all of the city's eighty-four police stations, Dr. Weinstein found an opportunity to tacitly revise his earlier description of smallpox. It was, he now declared, "the most contagious of diseases." He was rewarded on Thursday evening with word that half a million vaccinations had been performed during the day.

There was no perceptible letup in the public's desire for immunization during the remainder of the week, and on Sunday, April 20th, some additional interest was created by an announcement from Brigadier General Wallace H. Graham, the White House physician, that President Truman's preparations for a three-hour visit to New York the next day had included a brand-new vaccination. During the next week, two hundred Health Department teams, each composed of a doctor and a nurse, moved through the public elementary and high schools, vaccinating some eight hundred and eighty-nine thousand children. Toward the end of the week. Dr. Weinstein was sufficiently satisfied with the way things were going to reveal that the six surviving smallpox patients at Willard Parker and the four at Millbrook appeared to be out of danger. On Saturday, at his direction, the vaccinators were withdrawn from the police stations.

Six days later, on Friday, May 2nd, Dr. Weinstein formally announced the end of the outbreak and the completion of the biggest and fastest mass-vaccination campaign in the history of the world. Within the space of only twenty-eight days, he said, a total of at least six million three hundred and fifty thousand people had been vaccinated in the city. Practically everyone in New York was now immune. Although Dr. Weinstein had the delicacy not to say so, it was about time.

A Lonely Road

AROUND ten o'clock one September evening in 1934, a native of Puerto Rico, whose name shall here be Roberto Ramirez, was sitting at ease in the kitchen of his three-room flat on West 114th Street, a cigarette in his hand and a bottle of beer at his elbow, when he became aware of an odd and pungent odor. Ramirez, a married man of forty-one, with a nine-year-old son and a daughter of eleven, was alone in the room. His wife was out, at a movie with a neighbor, and the children were in bed and asleep. For an instant, Ramirez thought of fire. He cocked his head and sniffed. But the smell was not the smell of smoke and smoldering wood. It was more the smell of something cooking. It smelled like meat, like roasting meat — and it was. As he pushed back his chair to investigate, he saw it. It was his hand. His cigarette had burned away to a ruddy coal between the first and second fingers of his left hand, and the flesh for half an inch around was cracked and curling and darkly red. He dislodged the remains of the cigarette with a convulsive jerk, and stared at his wound. The sight of it made him shudder, but it might have been the hand of another man. It didn't hurt at all. Ramirez got up and went to the cupboard and smeared his fingers with lard. Then, in a panic of bewilderment, he sat down again and waited for his wife. Her consternation was anything but reassuring.

The next morning, still dazed with dismay, Ramirez presented himself at the general clinic of Harlem Hospital for a word of explanation. His confidence in medical science was not misplaced. The examining physician was neither greatly perplexed nor much perturbed. Loss of sensation, he explained, after inspecting the burn and modernizing its dressing, was not an unheard-of phenomenon. It could hardly be called even rare. It bespoke a neuritis — an inflammation of the nerves — and was more or less symptomatic of numerous ailments. They included tumors, certain deficiency diseases, and several bacterial infections. At the moment, the doctor went on, the evidence, though far from abundant, seemed to indicate that Ramirez's complaint was nutritional in origin. He suspected, he said, a chronic deficiency of vitamin B_1. If such was the case, the trouble was readily reparable. He then turned his attention from theory to therapy. He wrote out a prescription for thiamine hydrochloride, recommended a diet rich in milk and liver and whole-grain cereals, and advised a minimum of exercise. In addition, and as a matter of course, he exacted from Ramirez a firm promise to return in a couple of weeks for review and further instructions.

Ramirez was more than punctual. He was back at the clinic the following week. His burn was healing, but he had made an unsettling discovery. He thought the doctor ought to know. That morning, while washing, he had come upon a new, or at least another, patch of insensitivity. Like the first, it was on his left arm, but higher up, just above the wrist. He rolled back his sleeve and pointed it out. The spot he indicated was the color of parchment and slightly depressed. It was about the size of a quarter. The doctor gave it a long, reflective, and increasingly uneasy look. It didn't, he had to admit, much resemble the lesions characteristic of any deficiency disease. Nor was it strongly suggestive of any of the more familiar infections that had earlier crossed his mind. What it did resemble, he found hard to believe. He was astonished that the idea had even occurred to him. After a time, he stood up and stepped across the office to a tier of cabinets. He returned with a scalpel, a glass slide, and a carefully disarming smile. His explanation of his purpose was also shaped by discretion. There was a possibility, he said, that his original diagnosis had not been entirely correct. In order to make sure, he was going to extract a drop of material from the lesion for a bacteriological examination. It was a simple, bloodless operation, and took only a moment. Now, if Ramirez would just . . . exactly! He discarded his scalpel and held out a friendly hand. Analysis, of course, took somewhat longer. But Ramirez would be notified of the result in a day or two. Meanwhile, he was to continue as before.

When the door had closed, the doctor picked up the telephone and put in a call to the laboratory. He told the bacteriologist on duty there that he was sending along a skin scraping on which he wanted a prompt report. It was to be examined for acid-fast bacilli by the Ziehl-Neelsen method. Half an hour later, as he was preparing to duck out for a hurried lunch, the laboratory called back. They had received the scraping and it had been stained as requested. The reaction was positive. For a moment, the doctor was silent. Then he uttered a grunt of thanks, hung up, and reached for his pen and a piece of writing paper. The message he wrote was addressed to the director of the Bureau of Preventable Diseases of the New York City Department of Health. It informed him that Roberto Ramirez, male, of ——

West 114th Street, had been examined by the undersigned and found to be suffering from leprosy.

Of all the diseases that beset the human race, leprosy is by far the hardest to bear. It is usually disfiguring, it is often crippling, and it not uncommonly results in death. It is also chronic and contagious. In addition, it is incurable. What distinguishes leprosy from all other ailments, however, is not the progressive physiological dissolution that its victims must frequently endure. It is the fear and horror and violent loathing that it ordinarily excites in others.

The belief that leprosy unfits its victims for either the sympathy or the society of other men is supported by more than mere aversion. It has the sanction of Holy Writ. Both the Bible and the writings of Mohammed endorse it. "Run away from an Arabian leper as you run away from a tiger," the prophet advised his disciples at the beginning of the seventh century. Mohammed's inspiration, in this instance, was more derivative than divine. His attitude toward leprosy had been molded by an earlier prophet. The architect of lepraphobia was Moses. In the opinion of most medical historians, the universal abhorrence of leprosy is largely attributable to the heaven-sent dread of the disease that Moses communicated to the children of Israel. "And the Lord spake unto Moses and Aaron," the anonymous author of the Book of Leviticus records, "saying, When a man shall have in the skin of his flesh a rising, a scab, or bright spot, and it be in the skin of his flesh like the plague of leprosy; then he shall be brought unto . . . the priest. . . . Then the priest shall look upon it: and, behold, if the rising of the sore be white reddish . . . he is a leprous man, he is unclean: the priest shall pronounce him utterly unclean. . . . And the leper in whom the plague is, his clothes shall be rent, and his head bare, and he shall put a covering upon his upper lip, and shall cry, Unclean, unclean. All the days wherein the plague shall be in him he shall be defiled; he is unclean: he shall dwell alone; without the camp shall his habitation be." Moses received these explicit instructions some twelve or thirteen hundred years before the birth of Christ. Until then, lepers had been only informally shunned. Their good fortune vanished in the wake of the wandering Jews. Within a century or two, the intolerable impurity of the leprous had been sensed throughout the civilized world. The first full-dress demonstration of lepraphobia occurred around 1250 B.C., in Egypt. At the order of Ramses II, the monarch of the moment, eighty thousand lepers were wrested from their homes and resettled in a compound on the edge of the Sahara Desert. There is no record of how long they survived. The most recent display took place in China, in June of 1952, when the sub-prefect of a back-country province ordered approximately one hundred inmates of the local leprosarium burned to death. Three escaped the holocaust.

Leprosy probably originated in Egypt. It is possible that the Jews first encountered it there. There are allusions to an adhesive skin disease of catastrophic ferocity in many of the oldest Egyptian religio-medical writings, including the encyclopediac "Papyrus Ebers," which was assembled nearly four thousand years ago and is the most venerable manual of medicine in existence. "Papyrus Ebers" also suggests a remedy. "To drive away leprous spots on the skin," it reads, "cook onions in sea salt and urine, and apply as a poultice." The spread of leprosy from Egypt is indistinctly charted. It is certain only that it was among her earliest exports and that its advance in the beginning was rapid and easterly. By 1000 B.C., it was endemic in all of Asia. Its westward sweep, though eventually equally thorough, was somewhat less galvanic. It failed to get a foothold in Europe until almost the time of Christ. Leprosy was unknown to the ancient Greeks. It is, in fact, one of the few diseases of indisputable antiquity that Hippocrates neglected to describe. The introduction of leprosy into Europe is usually attributed to the legions of Pompey the Great. They acquired it, along with the treasures of Mithridates, during their triumphant tour of Asia Minor, and in 62 B.C. it accompanied them back to Rome. From there, in line of duty and in the course of time, they carried it on to Spain and France and Germany, and across the Channel into Britain. They also distributed it among the Greeks. To the Romans, the disease was known as "*elephas.*" The Greeks gave it its present name. "Leprosy" derives from "*lepros,*" an adjective meaning "scaly." The first reasonably recognizable clinical account of leprosy was composed by an Augustan aristocrat of scientific leanings named Aulus Cornelius Celsus. "In this [leprosy] the whole body becomes so affected that even the bones are said to become diseased," he noted, about the year 30 A.D., for the illumination of his friends. "The surface of the body presents a multiplicity of spots and of swellings, which, at first red, are gradually changed to be black in color. The skin is thickened and thinned in an irregular way, hardened and softened, roughened in some places with a kind of scales; the trunk wastes, the face, calves, and feet swell. When the disease is of long standing, the fingers and toes are sunk under the swelling: feverishness supervenes, which may easily destroy a patient overwhelmed by such troubles."

Celsus, though otherwise a sharp observer, seems not to have grasped the brutalizing quality of the new disease. His contemporaries were similarly obtuse. The Romans, like the aborigines of Egypt, were slow to develop an immoderate horror of leprosy. Its uniqueness had to be explained to them. Among the missionaries who contributed to their ultimate enlightenment, three are outstanding. One of these was the celebrated physician and teacher Aretaeus of Cappadocia. Aretaeus, who established himself in Rome toward the latter half of the second century, possessed a gift for portraying the serious side of disease that has almost never been equalled. His likeness of leprosy is generally considered his masterpiece. "The disease named 'elephas' and the animal named elephant have many properties in common," he wrote. "Formerly, this affection was called 'leontiasis,' on account of the resemblance between the disease and the lion, produced by the appearance of the lower part of the forehead . . . 'Satyriasis,' on account of the redness of the cheeks . . . 'Herculean,' because there is no disease which is graver and more violent. Its power is indeed formidable, for of all diseases it is the one which possesses the most murderous energy . . . also, it is filthy and dreadful to behold, in all respects like the wild animal, the elephant. Lurking among the bowels, like a concealed fire, it smolders there . . . [then] blazes forth . . . the respiration is fetid . . . Tumors prominent . . . The hairs on the whole body die prematurely . . . The skin of the head [becomes] deeply cracked . . . nose elongated . . . ears red, black, contracted, resembling the elephant . . . Sometimes, too, certain of the members of the patient will die, so as to drop off, such as the nose, the fingers, the feet, the privy parts and the whole hands; for the ailment does not prove fatal, so as to relieve the patient from a foul life and dreadful sufferings, until he has been divided limb from limb . . . libidinous desires [are] of a rabid nature. . . . Sleep slight, worse than insomnolency . . . neither food nor drink affords pleasure." Aretaeus concluded his study with a word of warning and advice. "There is also the fear that the disease may be communicated," he pointed out. "Many, for this reason, remove their dearest ones to solitude or to the mountains. Some preserve them from hunger for a time, others not at all, desiring their death." The other leading, if less overt, disseminators of the Oriental conception of leprosy were the apostles Peter and Paul. The Church of their founding was not based altogether on the compassionate gospel of Jesus. It also embodied the fierier teachings of Moses.

Lepraphobia and Christianity are closely linked. Both emerged from the ruins of Rome to sweep almost unimpeded through the Western world in the deeps of the Dark Ages, and both achieved their richest maturity during the long medieval twilight. The convulsive acceptance of the Trinity was everywhere in Europe followed by an equally convulsive aversion to the leprous. In 583, the delegates to the Council of Lyon, the first ecclesiastical convention held in France, unanimously approved a decree that prohibited lepers, under penalty of death, from fraternizing with any but their own kind. Their pious example soon fired the imagination of all wide-awake temporal authorities. Among the first to respond was an early ruler of Lombardy named Rothari. At his command, in 644, all leprous Lombards were seized and permanently sequestered in an abandoned building on the outskirts of Milan. Their support was left to the inclination of their friends. Pepin the Short, who was the father of Charlemagne and mounted the throne of the Frankish kingdom in 751, carried the Levitical ideas of his predecessors a step further. In addition to discarding his leprous subjects, he forbade them to marry, and declared that those already married could be divorced by their mates. Around 1000, during the reign of Olaf II, of Norway, who was subsequently canonized for his good works, the lepers of that country were simultaneously excommunicated, disenfranchised, and banished from all towns and villages. They were also pledged to celibacy. Olaf, a recent convert, was in one respect a trifle behind the times. By then, in the more civilized centers of Europe, it had become the custom to drive a leper into the wilderness only if he had the misfortune to be poor. Well-to-do victims of the disease were permitted, upon dividing their possessions between the Church and the Crown, to retire to a cell in a public asylum. At the beginning of the thirteenth century, according to Matthew Paris, a contemporary English historian, there were nineteen thousand lazarettos, as such retreats came to be called, in Europe alone. The term is of Biblical origin. It derives from a passage in St. Luke: "And there was a certain beggar named Lazarus, which was laid at his gate full of sores." One of the first English lazarettos was established in 1096, at St. Albans. A book of rules drawn up for the guidance of its inmates has been preserved. "Amongst all infirmities," the opening injunction reads, "the disease of leprosy may be considered the most loathsome, and those who are smitten with it ought at all times, and in all places, and as well in their conduct as in their dress, to bear themselves as more to be despised and as more humble than all other men."

In 1179, the Church introduced an additional mortification. It informed its deputies, by way of an ecumenical decree, that the banishment of lepers, while wholesome, was being carried out with offensive haste and informality. In the future, it continued, their separation from human society, instead of following immediately upon positive diagnosis by a physician (or, as was the custom in some places, by a magistrate), was to be preceded by a seemly religious service. The decree was accompanied by several sample ceremonials. "On [the] day [of exile], the leper must be clad according to his station, very simply," one of these, as elaborated by a twelfth-century French cleric, stipulates. "He must have on his head a white shroud, falling low behind, and a grave cloth over [his garments] and carry in both his hands a little wooden cross; and so move from his house accompanied by the church cross and by his friends mourning over him until he reaches the church. And when he has come to the entrance, the priest and clergy shall meet him and sprinkle holy water over him and take him by the hand and bring him into the cemetery and sing *Libera me Domine*. When they have come to the church, the priest shall begin the Vigils and the Commedaces, and when these are finished, the priest shall pray for him and say the Requiem Mass as for a dead man, with lights and candles. The leper, attired in his shroud and grave cloth, with his little wooden cross, shall kneel and lean on a low stool, his head bowed toward the altar — there where they are accustomed to place the bodies of the dead. And when the service is finished, the priest shall go to the leper, and read what is read to the dead, and then give him the holy water. Then the priest takes him by the hand, and when they are come to the cemetery, the priest makes him kneel, and throws earth over him three times, saying, 'Be dead to the world, and again living to God.' The priest shall then bless and present to the leper a hooded robe, a pair of gloves, and a bell to warn others of his approach, called the Lazarus Bell. He shall then admonish him: 'I forbid you ever to enter into church, abbey, fair, mill, or market, or into the company of others. I forbid you to go without your habit. I forbid you to wash your hands or anything about you at the stream or fountain, or to drink there, and if you need water to drink, take it in your cup. I forbid you to touch anything that you bargain for, or buy, until it is yours. I forbid you to go into any tavern, and if you want wine, whether you buy it or men give it to you, have it put in your cup. I forbid you to touch children or to give them anything. I forbid you to eat or drink from any vessel but your own. I forbid you to drink or eat in company, unless with lepers. If you go on the roads and meet another person who speaks to you, I forbid you to answer until you place yourself against the wind.' "

The wisdom of the Church in thus definitively demonstrating to the leprous their difference from ordinary pariahs was promptly and enthusiastically acknowledged by most medieval Christians. There were, however, in the course of the next hundred years or so, a few spasms of dissent. Several highly placed lepraphobes, including Henry II of England, his great-grandson Edward I, and Philip V of France, took the position that the recommended ritual was unnecessarily symbolical. The revisions instituted by Henry and Philip were similar. Both chose to replace the religious service with a simple civil ceremony. It consisted of strapping the leper to a post and setting him afire. Edward adhered a trifle more closely to the letter of the ecumenical decree. Lepers, during his reign, were permitted the comforts of a Christian funeral. Then they were led down to the cemetery and buried alive.

As a plague of pandemic proportions, leprosy reached its zenith in Europe in the thirteenth and fourteenth centuries. Its grip then suddenly slackened. It began to vanish around the middle of the fifteenth century. By the middle of the sixteenth, it was almost extinct. Numerous reasons have been advanced to account for its abrupt disappearance. Three are generally accepted. The unflagging zeal with which its victims were hounded and harried is, of course, one. Another is the several successive explosions of the Black Death, which, between 1347 and 1568, very nearly depopulated Europe. The third is the timely development of a diagnostic technique flexible enough to frequently distinguish from leprosy such other defacing afflictions as acne and scabies and scurvy. Of these reasons, the last is now widely considered the most persuasive. It is the current conviction of most authorities that only a fraction of the innumerable victims of medieval lepraphobia were actually suffering from leprosy.

Modern leprologists are capable to some extent of understanding the extraordinary horror of leprosy that haunted ancient and medieval man, but they find its present-day persistence peculiar. Any resemblance it may bear to reality is entirely coincidental. Leprosy is no longer obtrusively prevalent much of anywhere. Nor is it by any means the mystery it once was. Its source, its nature, and its clinical manifestations have all been pretty well fathomed. Nothing about it contains any unusual inducements to panic.

The cause of leprosy, which was determined by Gerhard Armauer Hansen, a pioneer Norwegian bacteriologist, in 1874, is a funguslike microbe of unparalleled sluggishness known as *Mycobacterium leprae*. Its lethargy approaches the comatose. Most pathogenic organisms make their presence felt within a week or two of arrival. A month is almost the limit. The incubation period in leprosy is rarely less than two years and it has run as high as thirty. Ordinarily, it is close to seven. The organism is also highly selective in its choice of habitat. Many parasites are able to adapt themselves to practically any physiological environment in a wide variety of animal hosts. *Mycobacterium leprae* can exist in no creature but man (all attempts to cultivate it in laboratory animals have failed), it much prefers men to women (the ratio is two to one), and it finds just two sites fully congenial. They are the under surface of the skin and the peripheral nervous system. When it lodges in the skin, the resulting infection is called lepromatous leprosy. Nerve involvement results in a type known as tuberculoid leprosy. Although the two types of leprosy may appear in conjunction, their characteristics are clinically distinct.

Lepromatous leprosy is the form usually envisioned by lepraphobes. It is marked by the gradual eruption on the face and hands and feet of a multitude of small, lumpy lesions that tend in cases of classic severity to grotesquely merge and ulcerate, and though its progress is slow, it ends nearly always in death. The life expectancy of a victim of lepromatous leprosy is approximately fifteen years. Tuberculoid leprosy is less conspicuously formidable. The lesions by which it manifests itself are macular, anesthetic, and somewhat resemble scar tissue. They vary enormously in size (from an inch in diameter to eight or ten) and they may appear on almost any part of the body. In a considerable number of cases, a few small blemishes remain from beginning to end the only perceptible evidence of the disease. In a majority, however, the destruction of nerve fibres is accompanied by some impairment of certain muscles, most often those in the fingers and toes. A few victims, in time, become helpless cripples. But, at worst, tuberculoid leprosy is merely disabling. It is very infrequently attended by pain, and it has never been known to be fatal.

Just how *Mycobacterium leprae* gains admittance to the

body is uncertain. Both the respiratory passage and the gastrointestinal tract have been suggested as likely portals. A third, and to many epidemiologists a likelier, possibility is that it enters by way of a bruise or laceration. But whatever the path to which it is partial, one thing is unequivocally clear. It can transfer itself from one host to another with only the utmost difficulty. Contrary to popular persuasion, leprosy is among the least contagious of all contagious diseases. In fact, under ordinary conditions its contraction is next to impossible. The disease is almost invariably, but by no means inevitably, a result of prolonged and intimate association with a lepromatous leper. Tuberculoid leprosy, to the best of medical opinion, is rarely, if ever, in any way communicable.

Although medical science has yet to find a cure for leprosy, the debilitating advance of the disease can often be hindered and sometimes even halted. There are several drugs to which it is more or less vulnerable. The oldest is chaulmoogra oil. Chaulmoogra oil, which may be administered orally, intramuscularly, or intravenously, is extracted from the seeds of a tree native to Burma. Its discoverer and first beneficiary, according to legend, was a leprous Burmese prince who happened upon it in time to return from banishment and claim his rightful throne. Chaulmoogra oil has been used in the Orient for a thousand years or so and in the West since the late nineteenth century, but because it is cruelly toxic and erratically effective, its popularity now is everywhere waning. The pharmacopoeia in current favor includes streptomycin, cortisone, and the sulfones. The last, which are distant derivatives of the sulfonamide group, are by far the most masterful. They were developed for general germicidal use by a team of British chemists in the middle thirties, but an American, the late Guy H. Faget, for many years medical officer in charge of the National Leprosarium at Carville, Louisiana, was the first to detect their value in the treatment of leprosy. Sulfone therapy was initiated at Carville in 1940. In 1947, after seven years of careful observation, Dr. Faget was able to report, "Experience has shown that the relation of improvement to duration of treatment [with the sulfones] can be approximately estimated. After six months of treatment almost twenty-five per cent of the patients show some improvement. After one year this percentage is increased to sixty, after two years to seventy-five, after three years to almost one hundred." Subsequent investigators have more than confirmed his findings. A large majority are fully satisfied that sulfone therapy, if continued for a minimum of three years, will result in at least some improvement in all but the most forlorn and fargone cases.

There are approximately four million lepers in the world. Around three million are concentrated in southeastern Asia, central Africa, and tropical Latin America. Most of the rest are widely scattered. The only considerable areas almost wholly free of leprosy are Canada and Siberia. It is endemic even in Iceland. In Europe, it is now largely confined to Spain, Portugal, Greece, Norway, Italy, and parts of the Soviet Union. Leprosy reached the United States, by way of the West Indies and the African slave trade, in the mid-eighteenth century, but it has never made much headway here. The American Leprosy Foundation estimates that there are at present not more than two thousand lepers in the entire country. Fully two-thirds of them, the Foundation estimates, acquired the disease elsewhere. Leprosy is endemic in just four of the forty-eight states — Florida, Louisiana, Texas, and, but only in its southern tip, California. Why this should be so has yet to be adequately explained. It is, however, demonstrably a fact. From time to time, cases of leprosy turn up in other states, but nearly all of them can be traced, directly or indirectly, to some foreign source. Four or five lepers, on the average, are discovered in New York City every year. In the fall of 1934, when Roberto Ramirez suffered his unsettlingly painless burn, the names of twenty-three local lepers were on file at the Department of Health. He brought the total to twenty-four.

The note from Harlem Hospital was handed to Dr. Samuel Frant, then director of the Bureau of Preventable Diseases and now Deputy Commissioner of Health, on Friday morning, September 25th. He gave it a long, unhappy look, added a few well-chosen words of instruction, and, as is usual in such matters, passed it promptly along to the Department's chief diagnostician, Dr. David A. Singer, for thorough investigation. Dr. Singer's reaction to Ramirez's plight was equally brisk and methodical. He tossed the report, the note, and a word or two of his own across to his secretary, and she typed out the customary letter. It read, "Will you please call on me at my office on Monday, October 1st, at 4 P.M. If you cannot appear at that time, kindly telephone my secretary and she will arrange another appointment." Dr. Singer signed the letter before he left for lunch, and it went out in the afternoon mail.

"Ramirez performed as expected," Dr. Singer says. "He didn't telephone and he didn't fail me. They very seldom do. They're afraid to. Our letter reads like a summons. They don't dare ignore it. It's too official. On the other hand, it very carefully says nothing that could possibly scare them away. Leprosy is a nightmare word. One hint of what we want to see them about, and they might simply pack a bag and run. That's happened. And, of course, you can't really blame them. They don't know any better. Most people are still living in the Middle Ages as far as their understanding of leprosy is concerned. Particularly of how we handle it. They still think in terms of quarantine and segregation — life imprisonment in a leper colony. In other words, a fate worse than death. Nothing could be farther from the truth. At least, in most parts of the country. Two-thirds of the lepers in the United States live pretty much like everybody else. Carville is for the very unfortunate few. And it's hardly a prison. It's a hospital — one of the finest in the world. The fact is only ten states — most of them, as might be expected, in or near the endemic areas — still insist on some form of isolation. Notification of the health authorities is the most required by law in any of the others. Most of us still feel that notification is desirable. But our reasons have changed a good deal. Up to a generation or so ago, the main idea was to protect society from the leper. That's only part of it these days, even in the Deep South. We're more interested now in the leper — in doing what we can to make his trouble more tolerable. Which includes protecting him from the ignorance and cruelty of society.

"Well, as I say, Ramirez showed up. He came in on Thursday at four on the dot. Obviously worried to death. I gave him a cigarette and we talked a bit and I got what I needed in the way of history. Born, raised, and married in San Juan, Puerto Rico. Moved to New York in 1929. A painter by trade. All very much as usual. At least forty per cent of our cases originate in the Caribbean area. Then I had a look at his arm. It was leprosy, all right — tuberculoid leprosy. Not that I'd had any serious doubts. A positive

Ziehl-Neelsen doesn't leave much room for argument. But, naturally, I like to see for myself. And I didn't merely look. I went over him from top to toe. Also, if only for the record, I took another skin scraping and some material for a nasal smear. Then I sat down and broke the news. I made it as easy as I could, but I told him the truth. All of it. There's no other way. I began with the report from Harlem, and went on from there. I told him what the test had showed, what leprosy is and what it isn't, and what we do about it — or, rather, what we don't do. I made that plainer than plain. That we had no intention of sending him away. That his life was no more over than mine. That he could continue to live and work and do pretty much as he pleased — for years, probably. And that no one would ever know but him and his family and us. All we asked was that he follow a few simple instructions, the first of which was to return the following week — same day, same time — for a talk about treatment. Then I went back and explained it all again. I won't say he took it with a smile. There were, as always, several very bad moments. But he took it. He finally came around. At any rate, he wasn't going to do anything rash. I was sure of that. You can generally tell. So we were over the hump. The rest, I had every reason to hope, was just a matter of time.

"I don't know when Ramirez broke the news to his family. Or how. That part of the business, thank heaven, doesn't often devolve on me. The job of telling the patient is painful enough. I waited a couple of days, until I could assume they had heard and thrashed it out. Then, on Monday, I sent a medical inspector up to the home for a good look at Mrs. Ramirez and the children. We don't very often find more than one case of tuberculoid leprosy in the same family.

But it happens. Offhand, I can think of five or six cases. So we always make certain. That goes without saying. Moreover, we like to see how our people live. It's only common sense to insist on the fundamentals of hygiene. Adequate toilet facilities, for example, and a separate bed for the children. By Thursday, when Ramirez came down for his second session, everything was well in hand. Nobody had sprung any surprises. As expected, our laboratory was in full agreement with Harlem. Both of my samples were unequivocally positive. The inspector's report was also unequivocal. Ramirez was our only problem.

"My second meeting with Ramirez was a good deal happier than the first. A week had done wonders for him. He had a good grip on himself and he couldn't have been more coöperative. Maybe his wife had helped. I met her some years later — a very sensible woman. But, however it happened, it was a big relief. They sometimes come back worse than ever. It all depends on how much nonsense they've managed to absorb. Nevertheless, I didn't take any chances. Leprosy is a lonely road. Even the best of them need plenty of encouragement. So I went over all the facts again and repeated all my promises. From there, I moved on to what we expected of him. It wasn't much. Certainly nothing very onerous. We wanted to see him at least once a year — my secretary would call or write — to evaluate his progress and make the usual tests. That was the major requirement. Of the others, the only one worth mentioning is this. He wasn't to sleep with or kiss or fondle his children. I don't mean to imply that they were in any real danger. Still, since children seem to be rather more susceptible than adults, it's just as well to play safe. I then took up the question of treatment. In those days, that meant chaulmoogra oil — an injection twice a week, administered by a doctor. He could get his shots from a private physician or at one of the several big public dermatological clinics. Just as he liked. My advice was the latter. As a matter of fact, I told him, I had talked to a man I knew at New York Skin and Cancer Hospital and arranged a tentative appointment for nine o'clock Saturday morning. He nodded. Whatever I said. And he meant it. He went. Around noon on Saturday, I called the hospital and checked. It wasn't necessary. I just thought I would. He'd been there, they said, and would be back on Wednesday. Well, that was that. He was on his way.

"During the next few years, I got to know Ramirez pretty well. I was seeing him twice a year here at the office, and every now and then I'd run into him up at Skin and Cancer and we'd stop for a minute and talk. We finally came to be something like friends. That's where I met his wife — at the clinic. As far as I know, he never missed a treatment. He must have had well over a thousand shots. I wish I could say they did him some good. But I doubt it. In fact, I doubt if chaulmoogra oil ever did anybody any good. The arrests we used to brag about were probably pure coincidence. Leprosy is very peculiar. It sometimes just plain peters out. Ramirez had no such luck. He was a better than average patient, but his case was fairly typical. Almost every time I saw him, I'd find a new lesion. By the end of 1942, or thereabouts, he had at least a dozen — all sizes — on his arms and legs and back. It could, of course, have been worse. Considerably so. For one thing, it didn't, as can easily happen, develop into an infection of the lepromatous type. Also, nobody ever knew — except, I suppose, his son-in-law. His daughter married — with our blessing — in 1944. She lives in Boston now. And his only disability was his left hand. Eventually, the first and second fingers — the site of the original lesion — became badly clawed. New lesions kept turning up, though. Six months or a year would go by and we'd begin to hope. And then there it would be — another. Until 1949. Two years before, in 1947, we started using the sulfones, and Ramirez, like all of our cases, was switched to that. At the end of a year, we couldn't be sure. There were no new lesions, but that had happened before. In 1949, however, we really had reason to hope. By 1950, we were sure. He was more than holding his own. There was actually some objective improvement. Don't misunderstand me. He wasn't cured. A cure for leprosy is still in the future. He wasn't even arrested. The samples I took at his second 1950 visit were still very definitely positive. But something had changed. Things were slowing down.

"There's no way of knowing what might have happened. No two cases are the same. Our 1950 meeting was the last time I ever saw him. Early in 1951, a few days before he was due to come in again, I had a call from Mrs. Ramirez. Her husband wouldn't be down. He was sick. He'd had a heart attack of some kind — it sounded like coronary sclerosis — and was up at Harlem Hospital. Apparently in very bad shape. The next thing I heard, he was dead."

A Pinch of Dust

AMONG the several reports and memoranda that came to the attention of Dr. Morris Greenberg, then chief epidemiologist of the Bureau of Preventable Diseases of the New York City Department of Health and now its director, on Wednesday, January 21, 1942, was a note initialled by the head of the Department's Bureau of Records. It was on Dr. Greenberg's desk when he returned from lunch. The message was short, explicit, and altogether flabbergasting. For a moment, Dr. Greenberg could only stare at it. Then he shook himself, picked up the telephone, and called his chief diagnostician, Dr. David A. Singer, who now heads the Bureau's Manhattan division. He told Dr. Singer that he had before him the names of six people whose deaths had recently been reported to the Department, and asked to be provided as quickly as possible with a full medical history of each. Five of the group — four females and a male — had died in Roosevelt Hospital, at Fifty-ninth Street and Ninth Avenue. Their names and death dates were: Bab Miller, December 29th; Juanita Jackson, December 30th; Josephine Dozier, January 1st; Ida Metcalf, January 3rd; and Charles Williams, January 8th. The sixth was a woman named Ruby Bowers. She had died on January 19th, at Bellevue Hospital. All were Negroes, all were unmarried, all had lived in or near the

San Juan Hill section west of Columbus Circle, and all were adults, their ages ranging from twenty-five to sixty-one. The cause of death was tetanus.

The abrupt thirst for knowledge that was excited in Dr. Greenberg by this generous set of coincidences was entirely understandable. So was his disconcertion, for tetanus is a disease of gothic ferocity. It has, however, one redeeming quality. It is not communicable. It is invariably the result of a wound into which a bacillus called *Clostridium tetani* has found its way. In the majority of cases, it is introduced by the instrument that inflicts the injury. Although the intestinal tracts of many animals provide a congenial habitat for *Clostridium tetani*, it is also commonly found in soil, especially that rich in manure. The adult organism, like many other bacilli, readily expires when exposed to air and sunlight, but the spores by which it perpetuates itself do not share this attractive trait. They are among the hardiest forms of life. Tetanus spores are impervious to most antiseptics, including the cruelest extremes of heat and cold, and, in the absence of the dark and airless environment that favors their maturation, practically immortal. They are also balefully abundant. Bacteriologists have encountered them on vegetables, in hay, hair, cobwebs, and clothing, in the dust of streets and houses, and even adrift in the air of hospital operating rooms. No wound is too small to admit a multitude of tetanus spores. In fact, the smallest wounds — abrasions and pricks and thready cuts — are sometimes warmly hospitable. There are two reasons for this apparent anomaly. One is that such wounds close rapidly and thus shield the mature or maturing organism from the withering touch of oxygen. The other is that they are nearly always ignored. The cause of tetanus is a toxin that possesses a shattering affinity for the central nervous system. Neither the chemistry of the toxin's generation nor the method by which it reaches its destination is fully understood, but its nature is no mystery. Five hundred times more explosive than strychnine, whose action it somewhat resembles, the toxin elaborated by *Clostridium tetani* is one of the most venomous poisons known to man.

Tetanus is the name generally preferred by physicians for lockjaw. They consider the latter more apt than adequate. The rigors of tetanus are by no means limited to an inability to move the jaw freely. Constriction of the masseter muscles is merely the characteristic symptom of onset. The physical manifestations of a fullfledged case of tetanus amply reflect the virulence of its cause. They are of such distinctive vigor and variety that the disease was among the first to be recognized as an entity. The accounts of clinical studies made by Hippocrates in the fourth century before Christ include one of a tetanus seizure that is still regarded as a model of acute observation. "The master of a large ship mashed the index finger of his right hand with the anchor," he wrote. "Seven days later a somewhat foul discharge appeared; then trouble with his tongue — he complained he could not speak properly. The presence of tetanus was diagnosed, his jaws became pressed together, his teeth were locked, then symptoms appeared in his neck; on the third day opisthotonos appeared, with sweating. Six days after the diagnosis was made he died."

Opisthotonous is a spine-cracking muscular spasm. Numerous physicians have been inspired to describe the appearance of a patient in opisthotonos, but a Cappadocian named Aretaeus, who conducted a wide and successful practice in Rome in the second century, is usually acknowledged to be its classic delineator. "Opisthotonos," he noted, "bends the patient backward, like a bow, so that the reflected head is lodged between the shoulder blades; the throat protrudes; the jaw sometimes gapes, but in some rare cases it is fixed in the upper one; respiration stertorous; the belly and chest prominent . . . the abdomen stretched, and resonant if tapped; the arms strongly bent back in a state of extension; the legs and thighs are bent together, for the legs are bent in the opposite direction to the hams." Not all victims of tetanus are called upon to experience the excruciation of opisthotonos. More commonly, though no less disastrously, the systematic paralysis that marks the disease is not accompanied by tonic convulsions. Sometimes, however, a spasm the reverse of opisthotonos occurs. Aretaeus's description of this form of tetanic attack is not only definitive but perhaps the most elegiac passage in medical literature. "But if [the sufferers] are bent forward," he wrote, "they are protuberant at the back, the loins being extruded in a line with the back, the whole of the spine being straight; the vertex prone, the head inclining toward the chest; the lower jaw fixed upon the breastbone; the hands clasped together, the lower extremities extended; pains intense; the voice altogether dolorous; they groan, making deep moaning. Should the mischief then seize the chest and the respiratory organs, it readily frees the patient from life; a blessing this, to himself, as being deliverance from pains, distortion, and deformity; and a contingency less than usual to be lamented by the spectators, were he a son or a father. But should the powers of life still stand out . . . the patient is not only bent up into an arch but rolled together like a ball. . . . An inhuman calamity! An unseemly sight! A spectacle painful even to the beholder! An incurable malady! . . . But neither can the physician, though present and looking on, furnish any assistance as regards life, relief from pain or from deformity. For if he should wish to straighten the limbs, he can only do so by cutting and breaking those of a living man. With them, then, who are overpowered by this disease, he can merely sympathize."

Aretaeus's melancholy view of tetanus has not been rendered seriously obsolete by the accomplishments of modern medicine. Tetanus, once its grip is fixed, is still an essentially incurable malady, with whose victims the physician can for the most part merely sympathize. A remedy effective at any but the earliest stages of the disease has yet to be devised; its treatment is largely confined to the prevention of complications and the moderation of pain, and surviving an attack precipitated by a large number or an undebilitated strain of *Clostridium tetani* is anything but likely. "The outlook in cases of generalized tetanus is always grave," Dr. Warfield M. Firor, visiting surgeon at Johns Hopkins Hospital, in Baltimore, has noted in a recent monograph. "Even in the best hospitals the death rate is frequently more than fifty per cent." In other than the best hospitals, and among those victims to whom no hospital care is speedily available, the death rate is seldom as low as fifty per cent.

Nevertheless, in most parts of the world, tetanus is no longer a very domineering menace. Not for some years has its avoidance been wholly a matter of chance. Since the late nineteenth century, when an extensive inquiry into the mechanics of the disease culminated, in 1889, in the isolation of *Clostridium tetani* by the Japanese bacteriologist Shibasaburo Kitazato, a prophylactic antitoxin (and, more recently, a toxoid that will confer an absolute and a reasonable durable immunity) has been within easy reach. Inoculation against tetanus is now compulsory in the armed forces of all nations, many business concerns throughout the world emphatically commend it to their employees, and in an increasing number of countries, among which the United States is outstanding, it is fast becoming an integral part of pediatric routine. For these reasons, and because most physicians are in the habit of administering a prophylactic charge of antitetanic serum whenever they are confronted by a suspicious-looking wound, the disease has been for nearly a generation — in this country, at least — something of a rarity. Its current incidence in the United States is hardly two thousand cases a year. Of these, on the average, only around fifteen turn up in New York City, and they are usually pretty well scattered among the five boroughs. Also, as might be expected from the solitary nature of the disease, they are generally far apart.

The clinical biographies commissioned by Dr. Greenberg on that winter afternoon in 1942 were compiled with the dispatch to which he is accustomed. They reached him the following morning, Thursday, January 22nd, at about ten o'clock. The first of the six on which he happened to fix his eyes was that of Charles Williams. "I visited Roosevelt Hospital today," wrote the operative Dr. Singer had assigned to the job, "and examined the records of Charles Williams. . . . History reveals that he [was] an old colored man, sixty-one years of age, and single. He was admitted to the hospital on January 4, 1942, at 7:00 P.M., with complaints of pain in the back of his neck for the past twenty-four hours and difficulty in swallowing for the past forty-eight hours. History shows that he was a [heroin] addict, having used injections into the skin for the past two years. On examination, the neck was rigid and his pupils reacted sluggishly to light. On January 4,

1942, he was given 100,000 units of tetanus antitoxin. On January 5th, he developed opisthotonos. . . ." Dr. Greenberg didn't bother to read any more of it. Instead, he turned to the next dossier. After a line or two, he let it drop, and glanced sharply at each of the others. A glance was all he needed. It was enough to convince him that he was indeed up against a series of related cases of tetanus. It was also enough to give him an excellent idea of how they must have originated. Like Williams, Bab Miller, Ida Metcalf, Juanita Jackson, Josephine Dozier, and Ruby Bowers had all been firmly addicted to heroin. Dr. Greenberg returned the reports to their folder with a somewhat muted sense of triumph. He was conscious that he had just made a vividly illuminating discovery but scarcely a reassuring one. If, as seemed probable, the six Negroes had contracted the disease from a common source, it might very well be one that was still accessible to others who happened to share their failing.

The task of determining the source of the infection fell to a field epidemiologist whose name, because he is now engaged in private practice and prefers anonymity, shall here be Ernest Clarke. He was not an arbitrary choice. Dr. Clarke was, and is, an investigator of some distinction in the field of tetanus, and it was Dr. Greenberg's expectation that the congeniality of the subject would supply him with an unusual and perhaps a rewarding zest for the task. He knew he would need it. Dr. Clarke accepted his attractive assignment with a rather clearer notion of what he was looking for than of where to find it. It could be anywhere in the warrens of San Juan Hill, and the only known people who might have been able to direct him were dead. On the other hand, he could conceive of just two possible vehicles that would be compatible with the evidence. A contaminated hypodermic needle was one. The other was a contaminated batch of heroin. At the moment, Dr. Clarke was inclined to favor the former. He was aware, however, that it really didn't much matter. One could hardly be less lethal, or elusive, than the other.

Before actively buckling down to the hunt, Dr. Clarke retired to his office and made a series of sedentary casts. At the end of an hour on the telephone, he was satisfied that nothing even suggestive of tetanus had been seen in the past few weeks at any Manhattan hospital except Bellevue and Roosevelt, and that if something, especially in a drug addict, did appear, he would be promptly informed. Then he dropped in at a restaurant around the corner and had a thoughtful lunch. From there, no livelier course having occurred to him, he headed first for Bellevue and then for Roosevelt. His retracing of the steps of Dr. Singer's agent did not imply a lack of confidence in the agent's ability as a medical historian. He merely hoped that his colleague, in a natural preoccupation with the clinical aspects of the outbreak, had overlooked some biographical detail that would give him a serviceable lead. If he had, Dr. Clarke was soon persuaded, it hadn't been at Bellevue. There was nothing whatever in the recorded history of Ruby Bowers that he did not already know. Still hopeful, though weighted by a new and discomfiting appreciation of his predecessor's thoroughness, Dr. Clarke moved on to Roosevelt. It was a little past two when he presented himself to the librarian of the record room there. He emerged from his studies at three, possessed of only one trifling nugget of additional knowledge. For what it was worth, he now knew that at least two of the six victims were linked by more than race, geography, and misfortune. Ida Metcalf and Josephine Dozier had been friends. During most of 1941, they had shared a room in a lodging house on West Fifty-second Street.

As Dr. Clarke rose to go, the librarian came hurrying over and asked if she could be of any further help. Dr. Clarke said he guessed not — unless, of course, he added wryly, she could conjure up another case of tetanus for him. The librarian gave him a reproachful smile. After all, she remarked, five cases in less than two weeks were — She stopped, looking stunned. As a matter of fact, she said in amazement, it was just possible, if sudden memory served, that she could. Then, sped by a stare from Dr. Clarke, she vanished into the stacks. When she returned, she had another folder in her hand. Dr. Clarke sank back into his chair, crossed his fingers, and opened the folder. Its subject was a woman named Lulu Garcia. She was colored, single, and fifty-three years of age. Her address was 530 West Forty-fifth Street. She had been admitted to the hospital on January 5th for observation, the findings of the examining physician having been provocative but inconclusive. They included headache, nausea, and a stiff jaw and neck. Also, the clinician noted in passing, she was plainly addicted to drugs. That night, the house physician took a look at her, and though what he saw failed to inspire even a tentative diagnosis, he prescribed a liberal dose of tetanus antitoxin. It was not repeated. There was no need. Nine days later, on January 14th, she was judged to be recovered from whatever had ailed her, and discharged. Dr. Clarke reached jubilantly for his hat.

At a quarter to four, Dr. Clarke bounded up the eroded stoop of 530 West Forty-fifth Street. At five, he slowly descended. He hadn't seen Lulu Garcia. She didn't live there any more. She had moved away a week earlier, and he could find nobody in the building who was able, or at any rate willing, to tell him where.

Dr. Clarke's withdrawal from 530 West Forty-fifth Street was only temporary. He was destined to become a familiar figure on the block. Two weeks later, he was still there and still stumped. He had by then had an endless monotony of conversation with every inhabitant of the building and with most of the people who lived next door or across the street. He had talked to the janitor and the rent collector and a dozen delivery boys. He had spent hours of inquisitive loitering among the loiterers in the corner stores and bars and lunchrooms. Twice, driven less by hope than by exasperation, he had made a long and garrulous tour of the other addresses on his list. But nothing had come of any of it. Lulu Garcia was not merely gone; she had vanished without a trace. Toward the end of the second week, Dr. Clarke sought out Dr. Greenberg for a word of counsel. Dr. Greenberg wasn't much help. He had nothing to recommend but persistence. The disappearance of Lulu Garcia, he admitted, was nettling, but, he added optimistically, matters could be a lot worse. The important thing, he reminded his colleague, was that she existed. Dr. Clarke began to wonder, as he glumly resumed his rounds, if she really did. A day or two later, on Saturday, February 7th, he received a telephone call that further tried his resilience. The call, which reached him at home and at breakfast, was from the medical superintendent of Harlem Hospital. He understood that Dr. Clarke had asked to be notified if a case of tetanus with evidence of drug addiction should happen to turn up at Harlem. Well, one had. The victim was a woman named Mildred Stewart. She was twenty-six years old, unmarried, and colored. Her home was on West 140th Street, and she had lain there, ill and alone, for several days. An ambulance summoned by neighbors had brought her to the hospital about an hour before. Dr. Clarke cut in with an impatient volley of thanks. He said he would be right up for a talk with her. The medical superintendent cleared his throat. That, he was sorry to say, would be impossible. The patient was dead.

Monday morning, February 9th found Dr. Clarke back on West Forty-fifth Street again. He had nowhere else to go. An active but uneventful weekend among Mildred Stewart's effects and neighbors had merely confirmed his belief that Lulu Garcia, in spite of her increasingly chimerical aspect, was probably still his only chance of success. It was about ten o'clock when he dropped off a crosstown trolley and made his way up Tenth Avenue to the familiar corner. As he stood there, trying to decide which of his usual haunts was the least hopeless, a man emerged from a nearby areaway, stared at him for a moment, and then raised a beckoning finger. He wanted to ask a question. Wasn't he the fellow who had been asking around for Lulu Garcia? Dr. Clarke took a deep breath and said he certainly was. Was he sure enough a doctor? Dr. Clarke produced his credentials. The man gave them an inscrutable glance. Most people on the block thought different, he said. They thought he was most likely a bill collector or a process server, or even a detective. He himself — he shrugged — he didn't know or care. But he saw no harm in doing a man a favor. It might come back to him someday. Bread on the waters. If Dr. Clarke was interested, Lulu Garcia had a friend or a relative or something named Mrs. Johnson. She lived at 417 West Fifty-second Street.

The house at 417 West Fifty-second Street turned out to

be a battered brownstone a few doors west of Ninth Avenue. Mrs. Johnson's apartment was on the fifth floor. A tall, robust woman of indeterminate age opened the door. Dr. Clarke introduced himself and, after explaining that his mission was both urgent and innocuous, said he was seeking a woman named Lulu Garcia. Mrs. Johnson, he understood, was acquainted with her. The woman gazed at him. Then she nodded, and stepped aside to let him enter. "Mrs. Johnson won't be back till later," she said. "But take a seat. I'm Lulu Garcia. What did you want to see me about?"

Dr. Clarke walked into Dr. Greenberg's office at dusk. Dr. Greenberg was just leaving, but at a provocative murmur from Dr. Clarke he discarded his hat, hung up his overcoat, and sat cheerfully down. "Congratulations," he said, and indicated a chair. "Which was it?"

"I don't know," Dr. Clarke said. "I've got a pretty good idea, though. Everything points to the heroin. For one thing, I'm satisfied that it wasn't a contaminated needle. It couldn't have been. Not if we believe Lulu, and I do. She has her own outfit. And so, she says, did Juanita Jackson and Ida Metcalf and Charles Williams. Charles Garcia, I should say. According to Lulu, that was his real name, and she ought to know. It seems they used to be married. And they were still friends. He and Lulu and Juanita and Ida generally took their shots together. The last time was at Lulu's place, somewhere around Christmas, just before they all got sick. And there's another reason for ruling out the needle theory. Lulu flatly denies knowing any of the others. And I believe her. Why should she lie? Why should she admit knowing Ida Metcalf, say, and deny knowing Ruby Bowers unless it was the truth? There'd be no point in it. But they're all linked up. Lulu didn't know Ruby Bowers or Bab Miller or

Josephine Dozier or Mildred Stewart, but she had heard of them — from Juanita Jackson. Juanita knew them all. She was what Lulu calls the runaround. They all got their heroin through her."

"And tetanus?" asked Dr. Greenberg.

"Yes, I know," Dr. Clarke said. "Juanita wasn't a real peddler. She just bought a little batch every so often, and resold it — what she could spare of it — to her friends. Well, one of those little batches was contaminated. I'm not entirely guessing. Lulu has an idea that the stuff they had at Christmastime looked different. Dirtier than usual, I gather. So it was probably cut. It was probably cut a good many other times, but I mean by Juanita. Hers was the one that did the damage. Otherwise, we wouldn't have had eight cases of tetanus. We'd have had dozens. I don't know what she cut it with, but you know how those addicts operate. They'll use anything that's handy. My guess is she mixed in a pinch of dust."

"I suppose that's as good a guess as any," Dr. Greenberg said. "Except for one thing. It doesn't explain why Lulu is still alive."

"I was coming to that," Dr. Clarke said. "As a matter of fact, it does. It's about the only explanation that seems to stand up. The last few times Lulu and her friends met, Lulu didn't get a regular shot. She didn't have any money for drugs. All she got, she says, was what she could cadge from the others. And they weren't overly generous. They only gave her just enough to keep her going."

Something Extraordinary

I SPENT a couple of hours one afternoon in the biochemical research laboratories of Chas. Pfizer & Co., Inc., one of the oldest and most considerable manufacturing pharmaceutical houses in the United States. There are Pfizer factories in Groton, Connecticut, and in Terre Haute, Indiana, but the company's principal establishment, an aseptic mesa of thirty-odd buildings that includes its entire research plant, is in Brooklyn, in the Williamsburg section. The business was founded there, in a pink brick building that is still thriftily in use, by two immigrant Württembergers — Charles Pfizer, a chemist, and Charles F. Erhart, a confectioner — in 1849. Their first product was a wormwood derivative called santonin, an essential ingredient at that time of medicines designed to eradicate intestinal worms. From that fragile beginning, the firm gradually expanded its facilities to embrace the manufacture of a robust line of basic drugs and chemical compounds (bismuths, mercurials, iodines, tartars, and the like) and the production, by a fermentation process in which it pioneered, of citric acid. Until about ten years ago, such drugs and chemicals, together with a select alphabet of vitamins, constituted the bulk of the company's output. Although their production is still both large and lucrative, they now account for just half of the firm's total earnings. The other half is derived from the manufacture of antibiotics. An antibiotic is a chemical substance generated by a microorganism, probably in the course of the metabolic process, that has the capacity to inhibit or destroy certain other microorganisms. Organisms that elaborate protective venoms of this sort abound in the turbulent microcosms of the soil. Every ounce of earth contains millions of them. Few, however, generate bactericidal material that is useful in controlling any of the numerous infectious diseases that hound the human race. Most microbial products are toxic, many are intractably volatile, and some are merely innocuous. Of around a hundred and forty more or less adequate antibiotic substances now known to science, only five are widely serviceable. They are penicillin, streptomycin, chloromycetin, aureomycin, and terramycin. Pfizer is one of the largest of all producers of penicillin and streptomycin, and it is the discoverer and sole producer of terramycin. It is, in fact the largest producer of antibiotics in the world.

The major source of antibiotics is the venerable family of parasitic and saprophytic plants known as fungi. Its members include smuts, rusts, molds, yeasts, mildews, and mushrooms. Nearly all fungi evolve bactericidal material of one sort or another, but that exuded by the various molds appears to lend itself most efficiently to therapeutic use. The curative properties of fungi have been sensed, at least dimly, for centuries. They are conspicuous in the folk pharmacopoeias of practically all races. The American Indian was aware of the efficacy of some varieties of mold, particularly those attracted to wood, as a wound dressing. Fungus therapy, like man, probably originated in the Orient. At least three thousand years ago, Chinese physicians were conscious that moldy curd of soybean had an ameliorating action on boils, carbuncles, and infected lacerations. In India, almost as early, a mushroom of the puffball species was recognized, not altogether mistakenly, as helpful in the treatment of dysentery. The ancient Egyptians were also familiar with the healing qualities of many fungi. The so-called Papyrus Ebers, an encyclopedia of ailments and alleviations that was compiled around 1500 B.C. and is the oldest medical work of consequence in existence, lists dozens of concoctions whose chief ingredient is mold or yeast. Some, such as an elixir of wood mold and brewer's yeast that is recommended for the correction of uterine displacement, are, at best, harmless, but most, particularly a wheat-mold salve designed to cure eczema, reflect remarkable empirical knowledge. Hippocrates thought well of fungi, especially yeast, which he advocated as a remedy for certain gynecological disorders. Another Greek physician, Dioscorides, who practiced in the first century, was satisfied that agaric, an edible and distinctly germicidal mushroom, possessed all the important characteristics of a panacea. The Grecian medicine chest was among the first of the Roman Empire's cultural acquisitions, and Pliny the Elder, in his "Historia Naturalis," devoted a chapter to mushroom druggery. "Perilous as they [mushrooms] be," he noted, "yet some goodness is in them. . . . They are employed as a remedy for the fluxes known as 'rheumatismi,' and for excrescences in the flesh of the buttocks, which they diminish and gradually consume. They also remove pimples and freckles on women's faces. Also, a wash is made from them, as is done with lead, to serve as medicaments for the eyes. Steeped in water, they are applied topically to foul ulcers, eruptions of the head, and bites inflicted by dogs."

As an empirical science, fungus therapy reached its apogee in Pliny's time. The frequently shrewd practical understanding of the peculiar powers of mushrooms and yeast and mold that the Greeks and early Romans managed to achieve was, until the past ten or fifteen years, never equalled. It was never even approached. Along with literacy, plumbing, and the monetary system, practically all comprehension of the clinical usefulness of fungi vanished from the Western world during the interminable collapse of Rome. Medieval physicians, though vivacious druggists, preferred less rustic remedies. With a myopic admiration for such restoratives as potable gold, eunuch's fat, and crocodile dung, they set an example that was followed by all save the most eccentric members of the profession throughout the sixteenth and seventeenth centuries. Even the gradual evolution, toward the end of the eighteenth century, of a pragmatic pharmacy did nothing to relieve the obscurity surrounding fungi. It was not until the third decade of the twentieth that any sustained medical interest in fungi was rekindled.

Although the prolonged eclipse of the fungus group is generally attributed to the difficulty with which scientific medicine was extricated from the credulities of the Middle Ages, its persistence beyond the nineteenth century was only in small part a result of medical floundering. It was chiefly a result of medical progress. The revelations concerning the nature of infection which resounded through the last half of the nineteenth century, notably in the work of Virchow, Pasteur, and Koch, encouraged several generations of investigators to emphasize the prevention of disease rather than its cure. The development of an arsenical specific for syphilis by Paul Ehrlich, in 1909, rejuvenated pharmacological research. It also set its course, not in the direction of fungi but, instead, toward the field of synthetic organic chemical compounds. There it might have remained had not chance, in the form of a laboratory accident, reacquainted the human race with the bactericidal vigor of fungi.

This providential mishap occurred one autumn morning in 1928 in the laboratory of Alexander Fleming, then director of systematic bacteriology at St. Mary's Hospital Medical School, in London. Fleming was engaged at the time in cultivating, for experimental purposes, a select assortment of pathogenic organisms, and it was his custom to begin each day with a parental glance at his charges. As he moved down the table on which the colonies were arranged, in the little coaster like glass plates known as Petri dishes, one of them, a culture of *Staphylococcus aureus,* caught his eye. In the center of it, sprung overnight from an airborne spore, sat a tiny thicket of a commonplace green mold called *Penicillium notatum.* "It was astonishing," Fleming has recalled, "that for some considerable distance around the mold growth the *staphylococcal* colonies were undergoing lysis [disintegration]. What had formerly been a well-grown colony was now a faint shadow of its former self. . . . I was sufficiently interested to pursue the subject. The appearance of the culture plate was such that I thought it should not be neglected . . . [but] I had not the slightest suspicion that I was at the beginning of something extraordinary."

Fleming was not, as it happens, the real discoverer of the antibiotic substance that he was subsequently to call penicillin. He was merely the first to pursue the subject. The Leif Ericson of bacteriotherapy was a nineteenth-century English physicist named John Tyndall. Tyndall caught a glimpse of the inhibitory abilities of mold, by way of a similar fortuity, in 1876. He was not unimpressed by the encounter, but he failed to comprehend its full significance. He laid the death of the bacteria to asphyxiation. During the next forty or fifty years, the phenomenon of microbial antagonism was observed, with varying degrees of perspicacity, by at least a dozen other scientists, including Pasteur, but none of them made much of it. Unlike Fleming, they were not sufficiently interested, or inspired.

Fleming's experience, which he presently and modestly recounted in the pages of the *British Journal of Experimental Pathology*, did not create an immediate stir. Progress again interfered. His discovery was overshadowed almost at once by the galvanic introduction of the first of the numerous sulfonamides. Nearly a decade passed before a band of British investigators, headed by Howard W. Florey, professor of pathology at Oxford University, were persuaded, largely by a closer reading of Fleming's contribution to the *Journal*, to buckle down to what turned out to be the first successful attempt to extract the antibiotic substance of *Penicillium notatum*, and three more years went by before they accumulated a large enough quantity of the drug for a definitive clinical trial. That monumental, if somewhat belated, triumph took place, again in London, in February, 1941.

The excellence of penicillin, like that of Ehrlich's magic arsenical bullet thirty years before, excited more than admiration. It also excited in a sizable body of American scientists an urgent desire to assay the germicidal potentialities of other molds. Their efforts were speedily rewarded. Streptomycin, which came to light in a spadeful of New Jersey soil, was introduced by Selman A. Waksman, professor of microbiology at Rutgers University and originator of the term "antibiotic," in 1944. Three years later, a group of Parke, Davis & Co. operatives discovered chloromycetin. Almost simultaneously, B. M. Duggar, an investigator in the employ of the Lederle Laboratories, came upon aureomycin. Terramycin, the Pfizer find, turned up in the summer of 1949. Although these five are, at the moment, the only antibiotics adaptable to ordinary clinical use, they constitute a far from meagre arsenal. Around forty per cent of all complaints that require the attention of a physician can be controlled by one or another of them. They are effective against every known rickettsial affliction — typhus, tsutsugamushi disease, Rocky Mountain spotted fever, and the like. They are effective against most infections of bacterial origin, including such monoliths of misery as lobar pneumonia, meningitis, gonorrhea, typhoid, undulant fever, plague, cholera, and, in the case of one — streptomycin — certain forms of tuberculosis. In addition, they are effective against two of the more unpleasant spirochetal infections, syphilis and yaws, and some viral disorders. About the only major infectious diseases of formidable stature that still resist antibiotic therapy are malaria, diphtheria, tetanus, botulism, smallpox, and poliomyelitis. There is no compelling reason to believe that even these will continue to do so for long. In fact, as I gathered during my tour of the Pfizer laboratories, it is not impossible that the present broad and energetic search for new antibiotics will lead within the next few years to the discovery of microbial antagonists capable of hobbling all infectious disease.

The president of Chas. Pfizer & Co. is a chemical engineer named John E. McKeen. Mr. McKeen, a native of Brooklyn and a graduate of the Brooklyn Polytechnic Institute, is forty-seven years old but looks about twenty, and he is short and sleek and restless. When I was shown into his office on the afternoon of my visit, he was prowling back and forth before a long row of windows, his eyes fixed on the ceiling, an unlighted cigar in his mouth, and a roll of blueprints under one arm. At the sound of my entrance, he halted and swung around. "Ah," he remarked, and, tossing the blueprints onto a table, moved rapidly across the room to greet me. It was a large and pleasant office, panelled in pine, hung with portraits and aerial views of Pfizer plants, and faintly scented with disinfectant. One of the portraits was a photograph of Alexander Fleming, inscribed "To John McKeen, with Kindest Regards." Mr. McKeen gave my hand a businesslike pump. "You're early," he said. "Good. There's plenty to see. The biochemical laboratory is a fascinating place. I'd hoped to be able to show you around myself, but I can't. Unfortunately, I'm tied up. Don't worry, though. It's all arranged. One of the other officers is going to take over. He'll be along in a minute. Meanwhile, let me introduce you to our founders." He waved a hand toward the wall. "Meet Mr. Charles Pfizer and his brother-in-law, Mr. Charles F. Erhart. Two great men. Mr. Pfizer is the gentleman with the muttonchop whiskers. He was the first head of this company. I'm the seventh. The second was that fine-looking old gentleman you see there on the other side of the door. John Anderson was his name, and he started out as Mr. Pfizer's office boy. He and I both came up from the ranks. I got my start as a control chemist. One among many. I don't believe anybody had more to do with the development of Pfizer & Co. as a grand old quality house than Mr. Anderson. Pfizer quality." He gazed at me. "The words are synonymous."

There was a sound of voices in the outer office. Mr. McKeen cocked an attentive ear. Then the door opened and a stout, pink-cheeked man of about fifty rolled majestically in. He had on a brown suit and a brown necktie, and he was smoking a slim brown cigar. "Gentlemen!" he said cheerfully.

"Hello, Jasper," said Mr. McKeen. He turned to me. "This is the gentleman I was telling you about. Shake hands with

Jasper Kane. Jasper is our director of biochemical research. Needless to say, he was a prominent member of the team that gave terramycin to the world."

Mr. Kane extended a rosy hand. "So was John," he said.

"After a fashion," Mr. McKeen admitted. "Off and on. Terramycin was quite a project. It cost us four long years and almost that many million dollars. Not that I begrudge a nickel of it. Or an hour. We were very lucky. We might have ended up exactly nowhere. That's research."

"You just cross your fingers and keep going," said Mr. Kane through a thunderhead of smoke. "Sometimes it pays off."

"In more ways than one," Mr. McKeen said. "One thing leads to another. I'll give you an example. Research has made this company one of the principal producers of citric acid. Our chemists have been largely responsible for all the major developments in that field. Well, that same research is what put Pfizer out in front of antibiotics. Commercial citric acid is a fermentation product. So are antibiotics. That let us in on the ground floor. When antibiotics appeared on the horizon, we didn't have to scramble around and start from scratch, the way most of the other houses did. We already had the basic know-how."

Mr. McKeen sat down on the arm of a green leather chair. "We got interested in antibiotics in 1941," he said with satisfaction. "In penicillin, I should say. That's all there was then. In a way, it was an accident. One of our fermentation chemists happened to come across an article on the subject in one of the British journals — the *Chemical Trade Journal & Chemical Engineer,* I think it was. Penicillin was still in the experimental stage productionwise. The method that Florey and Heatley and Chain and the rest of the Oxford school had worked out was not very promising from a practical standpoint. It was simply a laboratory technique. They hadn't had time to carry it any further. To give you an idea, their rate of recovery was approximately one part penicillin per one million parts of fermentation liquor. That isn't very stupendous. In fact, it's scarcely more than the concentration of gold in ordinary sea water. But they had shown that penicillin could be produced, and that was enough for us. With our knowledge of fermentation, it looked like our big opportunity. We set up an experimental production unit — what we call a pilot plant — over in the lab, and went to work. Then Washington stepped in. I needn't remind you that penicillin was a war product. There's no telling how long it might have taken to crack the mass-production problem if it hadn't been for the war. Five or ten years, at least. But the war provided the necessary impetus. We had to have penicillin and we had to have plenty of it and we had to have it fast. Washington put the best scientific brains in this country and England to work on it. They brought Florey over, and Heatley, and, eventually, even Fleming. At the same time, they rounded up the pharmaceutical industry. The first penicillin conference was held on October 8, 1941, in Washington. Three of us — Merck, Squibb, and Pfizer — came away from that meeting pledged to devote all our resources to the problem. In time, of course, the entire industry was enlisted, but we were in from the very beginning. Not only that. I'm proud to say that Pfizer was delivering penicillin to the government as early as the spring of 1942. However, it wasn't until 1944 that any of us really began to get results. That's when the basic production problem was finally licked. I say problem — actually, it was a dozen problems, but I'm not going to strangle you with technical detail. I'll leave that to Jasper." He smiled. "What it boiled down to was this — the development of a submerged fermentation process. Up to then, we had all been growing our mold on the surface of the liquor. That was Florey's method, and it largely explains why his recovery rate was so low. Surface fermentation utilizes only a fraction of the culture medium. Nothing could be more impractical. But there didn't seem to be any other way to grow the stuff. Mold requires oxygen. American ingenuity found the answer to the riddle. Submerged fermentation is possible because Pfizer engineers evolved a technique for aerating a liquid mass."

Mr. McKeen was silent for a moment. He plucked a bit of lint from his sleeve. Then he cleared his throat. "We've got a great deal to be proud of here at Pfizer," he said. "We're not resting on our laurels, though. That old American competitive urge won't let us. As long as there's a chance of finding one more antibiotic, you'll find Pfizer in there pitching. There's a lot of money in antibiotics. I won't pretend there isn't. But it's more than that. Streptomycin and penicillin and chloromycetin and aureomycin and our own terramycin are more than just commodities. They're more than drugs. They're life-saving miracles. When you can make a living by helping somebody else in the world, you've got a pretty good life." He stood up, stuck his cigar in his mouth, and held out his hand. "Or so it seems to me," he said.

The biochemical research plant turned out to be an inscrutable, block-square structure of eight stories directly across the street from the building in which Mr. McKeen and most of the other executives of the company have their offices. Mr. Kane set a leisurely pace toward it. A few steps from the entrance, he drifted to a halt and took a final pull at his cigar. Then, with a grimace of regret, he pitched it away.

"We don't smoke in here," he told me. "The only exceptions to the rule are the administrative offices, the washrooms, and the cafeteria." He swung the door open and led the way across a bleak rotunda to a waiting elevator. The operator was a muscular man dressed in white, like a hospital orderly. We lurched aloft. "I guess I ought to explain about smoking," Mr. Kane said. "The reason is rather important. It has nothing to do with fire. Practically nothing, anyway. As a matter of fact, the rule applies equally to eating candy. It's a personnel-safety precaution. A considerable part of the work here involves handling pathogenic organisms, and we don't want our people to have any occasion to be constantly raising their hands to their mouth. Of course, we have other safeguards, too — gloves and masks and so on." He smiled a reassuring smile. "Don't be uneasy. I'm not going to take you anyplace where there's the slightest danger. I can't. It's against the law."

The elevator stopped and we got out. We headed down a long white clinical-looking corridor lined with closed doors. The only sound was the reverberating clomp of our heels. Mr. Kane opened the last door on the left. "Here we are," he said. "Here's where everything starts. This is the mycology laboratory." I followed him into a labyrinth of marble-topped counters, ablaze with sun and laboratory glass — Petri dishes, test tubes, and stubby Erlenmeyer flasks. Moving purposefully about among the counters were three young women in white. One of them gave us a fleeting glance. "A mycologist sounds formidable," Mr. Kane went on, "but he isn't. I happen to be one myself. Mycology is simply the branch of botany concerned with fungi. In other words, this is where we screen samples of soil for microorganisms that look as if they might be capable of producing a useful antibiotic substance. I don't know whether you've ever read any of Waksman's papers. Waksman is responsible for a vast amount of basic work. Among other things, he pioneered in evolving the systematic soil-screening technique that we all use now. Well, his account of how he found streptomycin gives a very graphic picture of what we're up against. No one has put it more succinctly. He begins by saying he examined a total of ten thousand samples of soil. From them he obtained around one thousand individual organisms that appeared to possess some antibacterial properties. About one hundred of that thousand, it developed, could actually inhibit bacterial growth. Of the hundred, he was able to isolate just ten. The rest were too unstable. And of the ten, for various complicated reasons, only one proved to be worth bothering about. That was streptomycin. At that, he was lucky. The odds are steeper now. It's no longer enough just to find a new antibiotic. It has to be superior in some way — in strength, range, or lack of toxicity — to anything else on the market. We went through well over a hundred thousand samples before we hit terramycin. But terramycin wasn't the first antibiotic we hit. The first was streptomycin. So was the second. I guess we've rediscovered streptomycin at least a hundred times. Everybody has. It's quite common." He shrugged. "Only, Waksman got there first."

"Where do you get your samples of soil?" I asked.

"From all over," Mr. Kane said. "India, France, South America — everywhere. We have volunteers combing the earth for us. Airline pilots are among our best sources. And explorers. Whenever we hear of an expedition being organized, we get in touch with the leader. Most people are very obliging. Actually, it's no trouble. All they have to do is — Well, you might as well see for yourself." He stepped to a cabinet and pulled open a drawer, disclosing a litter of lumpy packets, each a trifle smaller than a postcard, and made of transparent cellophane. I plucked one out and looked at it. Clotted in a corner was perhaps a tablespoonful of what could have been powdered mustard. The name and address of the company was stamped on the face of the packet. On the back was a descriptive label. It read: 'P. C. Barbour. 20 March 1951. Mozambique, P. E. Africa. 17 Km. E. of Cheline."

I dropped the fragment of Portuguese East Africa back in the drawer. Mr. Kane chuckled. "It doesn't look like much, does it?" he said. "Just a dab of dirt. But appearances are deceiving. Actually, it's a universe. Every envelope in that drawer is crammed with living organisms — molds and yeasts and bacteria of all kinds. I guess *potentially* living organisms would be more accurate. Right now, they're in a dormant, or resting, state. They're spores. But given the proper environment, they will very rapidly resume their development, and mature and multiply. Microbiological analysis of soil begins with the providing of that environment. You can't learn much from a spore. They all look more or less alike, even under a microscope. A well-developed colony of microorganisms is something else. Most of them are not only visible to the unaided eye, as you'll see in a moment, but quite easy to identify. Soil analysis is a fairly complicated job. At any rate, it takes time. The first step is to separate into a number of relatively small groups the thousands of spores that are contained in every sample of soil. We do that by mixing half a gram of soil in fifty cc. of water. If you've noticed that girl up there by the window — that's what she's doing with all those flasks. She's making muddy water. That reduces the concentration of spores appreciably. When the soil in a flask has been thoroughly shaken up, we draw off a drop of the suspension — about five-tenths of a cc. — and smear it on a Petri dish containing a nutritive jelly of a sort known to favor the growth of most molds. Then we cover the dish to prevent contamination from the spores in the air, and put it away in the warm room to incubate. At the end of four days, we bring it out and take a look."

Mr. Kane paused, pushed the cabinet drawer to, and peered around the room. Then he touched my arm. "Down this way," he said, and struck off into the maze of counters. I trailed carefully after him along a narrow aisle flanked by hip-high hedges of glass. We emerged before a counter spread with a hundred or so covered dishes. "One of these ought to be enough to give you an idea," he said. "I'd hate to risk polluting something valuable." He reached out, hesitated, and then removed the cover of one of the dishes in the second row. I started. Thrusting up here and there from a sand-gray plain of jelly were a dozen fragile, cottony tufts of brilliant color. Some were as pink as apple blossoms, several were creamy white, others were green or orange or dandelion yellow. One was a dusty blue. It was an astonishingly beautiful sight. It looked like a tiny garden. Mr. Kane grinned. "Pretty, eh?" he said. "Unfortunately, that's about all you can say for this lot. They're all old friends. Most of those white colonies are yeast. The pinks are a variety of mold called Actinomyces. Some members of that family have produced our most valuable antibiotics. Most of them, as a matter of fact. That green one near the far edge is one the whole world knows. It's Fleming's *Penicillium notatum*. Of course, it's merely a curiosity now. Modern penicillin comes from a different strain, a far better producer. It's called *Penicillium chrysogenum*. Kenneth Raper, a Department of Agriculture man, discovered it in 1943, on a rotten cantaloupe he picked up in a market out in Peoria."

"What is that blue one?" I asked.

"Oh, that's a bug," Mr. Kane replied. "Probably one of the Salmonella. You know, the food-poisoning bacteria. They're pretty common. Which is one of the reasons why we don't smoke around here. To tell the truth, though, we don't come across a great many pathogens in the course of screening. Soil isn't the reservoir of disease that most people think. The vast majority of microorganisms are either beneficial or harmless. That's one thing. Another is that most of those that aren't seldom survive for long. About the only serious exceptions are the bacteria responsible for tetanus, anthrax, gas gangrene, and typhoid."

Mr. Kane slipped the cover back on the dish. "Well, that was about an average plate," he said. "Maybe a little under average. We can usually find something of interest. There are hundreds of different molds. Nobody knows how many. We're constantly turning up new ones. Or what look like new ones. Some varieties are impossible to identify until you've seen them in action. Anything that looks at all promising, we isolate for thorough study. None of the girls seem to be working on that phase right now, but no matter. It's easy enough to describe. We simply pick off the colony we want with a sterile needle, drop it into a test tube of jelly, and return it to the warm room for a second period of growth. After about a week, we make another transfer. You can't extract an antibiotic substance from a solid medium. But, as Florey demonstrated, you can from a liquid. So we remove the culture from the tube to a flask of nutrient broth. Then it goes back to the incubator for two or three days or more, depending on its growth rate. Some molds mature faster than others. Then the bacteriological assay laboratory takes over. That's where the cultures are tested for antibiotic activity. I want you to see how we do that. Then we'll have a look at the pilot plant." He raised an immaculate cuff and glanced at his watch. As we moved back up the aisle, he added, "I don't mean to imply that the pilot plant is the last step. It isn't. A good many antibiotics get that far and still eventually come to nothing. Some turn out to be old friends in disguise. Some turn out to be too toxic. Some turn out to be just plain incapable of functioning in living tissue. They're marvels in vitro but worthless in vivo. But the pilot plant is as far as I can take you. Everything beyond that stage is restricted, for reasons of sterility or safety."

Two long corridors and a flight of stairs brought us to the office of the bacteriology laboratory. It was a small, tidy room, walled with filing cabinets and furnished with two desks. Behind one of the desks, a young woman was working at a typewriter. She looked up as we entered. "Oh!" she said. "Good afternoon, Mr. Kane. I'm afraid Dr. English isn't . . . Is there anything I can do?"

Mr. Kane resettled her with a genial shake of his head. "We're just wandering around," he said. Skirting the deserted desk, he led me through an inner door, down a short passage, and into a bright, stark, windowless chamber. On the wall, just to the right of the door, hung a framed certificate, signed and sealed by the New York City Department of Health. It read, in part: "Registration of Premises to Handle or Cultivate Live Pathogenic Microorganisms or Viruses." A massive worktable, on which were deployed a number of lidded Petri dishes, stood in the middle of the room. Above it was suspended an angular chandelier of ultraviolet germicidal lamps.

Mr. Kane removed the cover from the nearest dish. In the center, surrounded by a film of jelly, lay a paper disc about the size of a dime. Radiating out from the disc to the rim of the plate, like the spokes of a wheel, were six shallow indentations a trifle darker in color than the jelly. They looked as if they might have been scratched there with the charred end of a match. Mr. Kane gave a grunt of mild disgust. He pushed the dish aside and uncovered another. "Well, that's more like it," he said. "Quite a difference, isn't there?" I nodded. There was. In the second dish, the shadowy spokes were less clearly defined. Only three of the six extended all the way from the disc to the rim. Two of them ended abruptly half an inch or so from the disc. The other had almost vanished.

"What happened?" I asked.

"Antibiosis," he said. "The first, of course, was a dud. Here's how it works. It's really quite a simple test. As you can see, the procedure isn't unlike the one we use in plating out soil samples. Only, in this case we inoculate the medium with bacteria. That's what those ditches are. They're cultures of different pathogens. The kind depends on what diseases we happen to be interested in at the moment. If we're looking for an antibiotic of potential usefulness against tuberculosis, we'll use a selected strain of *Mycobacterium tuberculosis,* and so on. I don't know just what things English is testing for right now — they vary from time to time — but a representative selection might include the typhoid organism, one of the staphylococci, something in the field of urinary-tract infection, a pneumococcus, a meningococcus, and possibly a *Hemophilus pertussis,* the whooping-cough bug. As you probably know, those are all bacteria. The test for antiviral activity are run off in another laboratory. They involve the use of infected chick embryos instead of plate cultures, but I'm not going to attempt to describe them. They're much too complicated. The same goes for the rickettsiae, only more so. In addition, they're extremely risky. We don't even do them. No house does. All our screening for rickettsial activity is done for us by the Harvard Medical School. But to come back to bacteriology. When the bacterial cultures are well established, we dip a round of filter paper — one of those discs there — in a flask of broth containing a mature growth of mold and set it out on the dish. If the mold is capable of producing an antibiotic, it will be present in the broth, and the filter paper will soak up all we need. That's one of the most remarkable characteristics of an antibiotic — its high specific activity. Of course, to be effective, all drugs must be able to withstand a good deal of dilution without loss of potency. But the antibiotics are unique in that respect. Some organisms are sensitive to some antibiotics in solutions containing as little as one part antibiotic to one hundred million parts of diluent. That's what makes a test like this possible. Otherwise, the almost immeasurably minute amount of antibiotic substance present in that little disc could never have had the effect you see on the cultures in those three ditches. One culture practically wiped out and two very definitely inhibited. Unfortunately, a sight like that is pretty rare. Only about five per cent of our molds show any promising kind of antibiotic activity. The rest turn out exactly like that other — nothing." He picked up the covers and fitted them back on the dishes. "As a matter of fact." he added, "even some of those that do show some activity never get to the pilot plant. Biochemical analysis always eliminates a few of them. They just won't lend themselves to any kind of practical production."

We were still some distance from the pilot plant, moving down another lifeless corridor, when I caught a whiff of something sweet and damp and musty. It was a familiar smell, but for a moment I couldn't place it. Then, as we approached a heavy door at the end of the corridor, the smell grew stronger, and I remembered. It was the dark, earthy smell of a country cellar in summer. Mr. Kane saw me wrinkling my nose, and smiled. "Mold," he told me. "Or, rather, a combination of mold and broth. What you're actually smelling is fermentation. If you think this is powerful, you ought to walk by one of our main production buildings. You'd swear you were passing a distillery. A couple of months ago, a tenement over that way burned down. In the ruins, the police found the remains of a still. All the neighbors had smelled it — you can't disguise the smell of an operation like that — but apparently nobody had given it a thought. They thought it was penicillin."

Mr. Kane laughed. He opened the door, releasing a blast of pungent warmth, and waved me into a glitter of white tile, reptilian pipes, and polished metal tubs — huge, hooded, and wholly enigmatic — patrolled by a squad of men in spotless white. Several of the men had writing boards under their arms, and one was crouched at the base of a tub, staring at a panel of dials and making an occasional note. At the far end of the room, silhouetted against a wall of windows, rose three great cylindrical tanks of stainless steel. They were at least twenty feet high and perhaps five in diameter, and each was capped by a bristling growth of pipes and gauges and levers and wheels. Girdling the three tanks.

some fifteen feet above the floor, was a narrow, railed catwalk, reached by an iron stairway. We emerged from the parade of hulking tubs at the foot of the stairs. "You don't often see fermentation tanks this size in a pilot plant," Mr. Kane said, heaving himself agilely up ahead of me. "They'll hold two thousand gallons apiece. The average is around three hundred. But, compared to the tanks we use in commercial production, they're pygmies. We've got some up at Groton with a capacity of twenty-five thousand gallons. However, that's the only difference — size. These tanks and the biggest ones all operate on the same principle. John McKeen gave you a rough idea of how submerged fermentation works. If you remember, he said it involved aerating a liquid mass. Well, the air is introduced into the broth by means of a high-pressure sparger in the base of the tank. Sterile air, of course. But there's more to the problem than that. Left to itself, the mold would naturally tend to accumulate on the surface of the broth. We prevent that by a system of agitators fixed to a central vertical shaft. They keep the mass in a turmoil, and the result is growth at every level. Maybe you'd like to take a look." He indicated a small glass porthole set in the shoulder of the nearest tank. I rubbed away a film of moisture and peered in. At first, I could see nothing but darkness. Then the darkness dissolved into a murky twilight, and I could just make out a tiny fury of sand-colored foam. There was nothing else. "Disappointed?" Mr. Kane asked as I straightened up. "I always am. Too much like a washing machine."

"How much antibiotic does a tank this size produce?" I asked.

"That depends," Mr. Kane replied. "It's largely up to the mold. As you know, some are heavier producers than others.

We'll seed one of these tanks with anywhere from two ounces to five gallons of pure culture. The incubation period varies, too. A few molds will produce their maximum of antibiotic in a couple of days. Others need a week. I'd say the average return from a two-thousand-gallon tank is about nine pounds. We don't necessarily recover that much, though. There's almost always some loss during extraction. Those machines down there on the floor are all extractors of one kind or another. I'm going to give you the simplest possible notion of that phase of our operation. The procedure is roughly this: When the antibiotic has been excreted into the broth, we pump the whole mass of material out of the tank and through a rotary drum filter. That separates the liquor from the mold. Then the mold is discarded and the liquor is piped through a series of centrifugal extractors, each containing a different chemical solvent, which eliminates by absorption certain extraneous matter. At the end of six or seven passages, we're left with a fairly pure concentrated solution of antibiotic and water. We run that through another filter, this time for the purpose of sterilization, and then into an evaporation tank. The result is a bucket of more or less colorless crystals. It's also either the end or the beginning. That's when we find out what we've got."

We were standing at the catwalk rail, looking down at the men and machines on the floor below. For a moment, neither of us spoke. Then Mr. Kane turned toward the stairs. As we passed the tank whose contents I had glimpsed, he put out a hand and lightly brushed its flank. It was an odd, caressing gesture. "You never know," he said. "All you can do is hope. We seeded this tank this morning with a mold that — well, to put it mildly, it looks like a wonder. It looks even bigger than terramycin. In other words, it's just possible that with fifty-seven million square miles of earth to choose from, we've been lucky enough to pick up the prize handful. But, as I say, you never know." He gave me a rueful smile. "It's also very possible," he said, "that all we've done is rediscover streptomycin."

Family Reunion

TOWARD dusk on Friday, November 25, 1949, the day after Thanksgiving, a forty-year-old resident of Craryville, Columbia County, New York, whom I will call Charles Pappone, was helped by his wife and their teen-age daughter into the receiving room of the Albany Hospital. Pappone needed help. His head was splitting, his legs were like water, and his vision was blurred and failing. Also, he informed the examining physician in a gravelly croak, there seemed to be something wrong with his throat. It wasn't exactly sore. It just felt stiff and tight. In fact, it was almost impossible for him to speak at all. His wife anxiously took over. The trouble had started the night before, she explained. They had driven down to New York for Thanksgiving dinner with her parents, and on the way back to Craryville her husband had begun to complain about feeling weak. Then his eyes began to bother him. By the time they reached home, everything looked fuzzy. And this morning, all of a sudden, he had started to see double. She had tried to get their doctor, but he was out on calls. Finally, they had become frightened. There had been so much polio going around all fall. The papers said it was the worst epidemic in years. But, of course, it couldn't be that. Or could it? The examining physician shrugged. At the moment, he said, reaching for an admittance form, it was hard to say. He spoke with more compassion than candor. The opinion he was inscribing on the record read, "Suspected poliomyelitis."

Pappone passed a peaceful night in the hospital. The following day, he lay like a log, but he seemed at least no worse. His temperature, which had been normal at the time of his admittance, still held steady, and while neither his voice nor his vision had improved, his mind remained clear and he was altogether free from pain. Even his headache had gone. But on Sunday, at breakfast, a new trouble appeared. After one sip of orange juice, he had to stop. It was more than he could do to swallow. The muscles in his throat felt dead. An hour or two later, he was breathing hard, and choking on his own saliva. The nurse summoned an interne. He arrived on the run with a suction tube. Presently, having drawn off the worst of the congestion, he administered an eruptive dose of ipecac. Pappone's relief was immediate, but it was not of long duration. When the attending physician stopped by on his morning patrol, the patient was again gasping for breath. One good look was all the doctor needed. It showed him a perceptibly progressive paralysis that was beginning to involve the entire upper respiratory system. The doctor's instructions were, under the circumstances, conventional. They included a prompt tracheotomy (the making of an artificial opening in the windpipe), the use of a mechanical respirator, and a regimen of intravenous feeding. He also requested a lumbar puncture. A lumbar puncture is made for the purpose of analyzing the chemical and cellular composition of the cerebrospinal fluid and is, among other things, a generally reliable laboratory aid in establishing a diagnosis of poliomyelitis. Although the attending physician had earlier seen no reason to challenge his colleague's reading of the case, it now struck him as a trifle shaky. Pappone's unexpected decline distorted the clinical picture. In poliomyelitis, the doctor was uncomfortably aware, such violent turns are usually foreshadowed by some degree of pain and fever.

When the attending doctor reached the hospital on Monday morning, the report from the laboratory was on his desk. He read it, reread it, and tossed it aside. The report was negative. Pappone's spinal fluid was normal. This gave the doctor, however, no urge to exult. He had merely escaped from error into doubt. The doctor sat down and reflected. He emerged from his meditations with the feeling that just two possibilities were compatible with the evidence. One of them was epidemic encephalitis. The other was a form of food poisoning called botulism. He looked again at the laboratory report. It didn't precisely support either one, but it rendered the former the more unlikely. Encephalitis, like poliomyelitis, seldom fails to create at least a minor disturbance in the spinal fluid of its victims. The doctor took a deep breath. Then he picked up the telephone and dialled the laboratory of the State Department of Health. He asked the laboratory to provide him at once with thirty thousand units of therapeutic botulinus antitoxin.

Food poisoning is among the commonest of ailments. It is almost as common as the common cold and, in general, only a little less innocuous. It is also about as widely misunderstood. As a source of wild fears and wilder temerities, it is practically unequalled in the popular mythology of medicine. The most durable delusion in connection with it is that the great majority of acute gastrointestinal upsets are a result of ptomaine poisoning. Even doctors sometimes succumb to this fancy. "In one series of forty-three fatal cases in which the reported diagnosis was ptomaine poisoning, necropsy revealed in every instance some other cause of death," Dr. Walter C. Alvarez, of the Mayo clinic, noted in a recent study. "[These causes included] appendicitis, ruptured ectopic pregnancy, peritonitis, tuberculosis, meningitis, encephalitis, acute alcoholism, carbon-monoxide or metallic poisoning, toxemia of pregnancy, abortion, malaria, diphtheria, fulminating poliomyelitis, bacillary dysentery, coronary disease, pneumonia, and cerebral apoplexy." The diagnosticians involved, as Dr. Alvarez saw no need to add, were doubly deluded. Ptomaine poisoning is a product of the imagination of a nineteenth-century Italian toxicologist named Francesco Selmi. Selmi announced the existence of what he called ptomaines in 1870. They were, he explained to an attentive medical world, noxious substances generated in numerous foods in the natural course of putrefaction. By and large, he added, food poisoning and ptomaine poisoning were synonymous. Selmi was for many years a towering figure in medicine, but his stature has lately shrivelled. About the best that can now be said for his theory is that the name he gave it was an apt one. "Ptomaine" derives from "*ptōma*," the Greek for "corpse" or "carcass." Modern investigators are far from convinced that any such thing as a ptomaine exists. In any event, they point out, it could have no relation to food poisoning. Age alone has nothing whatever to do with the wholesomeness of food. Its irrelevance has been demonstrated by chemical analysis, by experiments with laboratory animals, and by millions of Chinese lovers of rotten eggs, Eskimo lovers of putrefied fish, and Western lovers of overblown cheese.

The nature of food poisoning has been pretty well riddled since Selmi's time. Clinicians now recognize three major types. Their sources are clearly distinct. One is food contaminated with some pernicious inorganic chemical. Inherently poisonous plants or animals (certain mushrooms, rhubarb leaves, some yams if eaten raw, faba beans, many tropical fish, and, at seasonal intervals, Pacific clams and mussels) are, of course, another. The third is food made toxic by the presence of certain pathogenic bacteria. Of the three, the first is probably the most unreasonably dreaded. Cooks have been known to mistake roach powder (sodium fluoride) for baking soda, or rat poison (barium carbonate) for flour, but such blunders are rare to the point of freakishness. Moreover, even when they occur, the consequences are by no means always catastropic. Chemical poisoning more often than not provides its own antidote. Usually its victims are at once convulsed by a salubrious fit of vomiting. Most fears of chemical poisoning are wholly hallucinatory. Contrary to nearly universal assumption, there is no conclusive evidence that illness is the invariable result of eating fruit sprayed with lead arsenate or any other conventional insecticide. "Lead arsenate ingested as spray residue [was] not accompanied by . . . the occurrence of any clinical findings," a United States Public Health Service Bulletin recently reported at the end of a three-year study of nearly two hundred and fifty orchard workers who habitually ate unwashed apples and pears. Nor, as many people persist in believing, is the use of aluminum cooking utensils a possible source of illness. Aluminum far from being a poison, has a respected place on the modern medicine shelf. One form, aluminum hydroxide, is widely considered the drug of choice in the treatment of peptic ulcer. Tin is also prominent in the toxicology of hearsay. Its inclusion is entirely undeserved. "Tin, in the amounts ordinarily found in canned foods and in the quantity which would be ingested in the ordinary individual diet, is for all practical purposes eliminated and is not productive of harmful effects on the consumer of canned foods," the Bureau of Chemistry and Soils of the Department of Agriculture has reported. A hardy corollary of the distrust of canned food, and perhaps the deepest-rooted of all such over-anxieties, is the belief that food should never be left in an opened can. "This [belief] is a myth of long standing," Dr. Gail M. Dack, professor of bacteriology at the University of Chicago and director of its Food Research Institute, has noted in an authoritative monograph. "Spoilage results from bacteria growing in a food, and, once the food is contaminated, time and suitable temperature will cause spoilage, regardless of whether the food is in a tin can or in a glass or porcelain dish. In fact, contamination is less likely to occur if the food is left in the can." The can, Dr. Dack went on to point out, is more apt to be sterile than the dish.

The usual cause of food poisoning is bacteria. Bacteria of one kind or another are responsible for well over ninety per cent of all outbreaks. The amount of misery these organisms inflict on the human race is incalculable. Everybody has felt their enfeebling touch at least once, and people who frequently eat in restaurants have experienced it numerous times, though not always with clear recognition. One is often only vaguely conscious of their presence. Many epidemiologists believe that most momentary indispositions whose chief characteristic is an uneasy stomach or a spasm of diarrhea are of bacterial origin. The vast majority of attacks are the work of any one of three varieties of bacteria — the staphylococci, the streptococci, and the salmonellae. All are sturdy, prolific, and ubiquitous. Each has its distinguishing traits, but from a practical public-health standpoint staphylococcal, streptococcal, and salmonellal food poisoning are all pretty much the same. They are equally abrupt, equally mild and of equally short duration, and, despite the reassurance of common sense, equally difficult to dodge. Their avoidance is entirely a matter of luck. The presence in a food of even a multitude of such pathogens can be detected solely by laboratory analysis. They in no way alter its appearance, its odor, or its taste. Nor, for the most part, do any of the several other microbes or microbial products that are an occasional cause of food poisoning. The only notable exception to this insidious rule is a toxin elaborated by a bacillus called *Clostridium botulinum*. Botulinus toxin is the cause of botulism. Food into which a lively colony of *Clostridium botulinum* has found its way sometimes emits a disgusting smell. Providentially, it is a distinctively disgusting one. Between 1899 and 1947, according to a compilation by Dr. Karl F. Meyer, director of the George Williams Hooper Foundation for Medical Research at the University of California, only twelve hundred and fifty-three cases of botulism were reported in the whole of the United States and Canada. Of them, however, eight hundred and fifteen, or approximately sixty-five per cent, were fatal.

Botulism is a true but atypical form of food poisoning. Its methodical approach, its excessive lethality, and the predominantly neural cast of its clinical features all are unpleasantly peculiar. Even its history is unusual. Ordinary food poisoning, in common with many other ailments, is probably as old as mankind. Its beginnings go back to the first butcher with an infected finger, the first cook with a streptococcic cough, the first imprudent assumption of the first man rash enough to eat mushrooms. Botulism is of far less fundamental origin. It is, in fact, one of the very few diseases for whose existence man has nobody to blame but himself. Like carbon-monoxide poisoning, and alcoholism, and the bends, botulism is essentially, if inadvertently, a product of human ingenuity. *Clostridium botulinum,* though plethorically abundant throughout the world, is not among man's natural antagonists. The organism is incapable of establishing itself in any living plant or animal. Its home is soil and earthy dust, its food is inanimate matter, and although it is able to exist in a dormant, sporal state almost indefinitely in almost any environment, it can mature and multiply and manufacture its vigorous venom only in the total absence of oxygen. Because of these physiological quirks, the toxin of *Clostridium botulinum,* under normal conditions, is safely out of human reach. It is dissipated deep in the earth. Exactly when botulism seized its first victim is unknown, but it could hardly have been more than eight or ten thousand years ago, when man ceased to subsist exclusively on fresh food. Freshly gathered food, along with everything else on the face of the earth, is exposed to the intrusion of dust-borne botulinus spores, but it is also exposed to the spore-stunting sweep of air. Botulism came into being when man made the otherwise triumphant discovery that prompt deoxidation would make numerous foods more or less permanently resistant to decay.

Despite the profusion of potentially hospitable harbors created by man for wandering *Clostridium botulinum* (canned or pickled fruits and vegetables, and canned, smoked, or pickled meats and fish and poultry), botulism has never been a very broadly urgent problem. There is no good reason why it should be. This is not, as might be supposed, entirely because of the repellent odor that the active organism may impart to its habitat, for the warning reek is not always present. Certain foods may be saturated with botulinus toxin and still smell much as usual. One of the most important determining factors appears to be the *p*H, or relative acidity, of the food. As a rule, the smell is most pronounced in non-acid foods — in meat, for example, and fish. Among acid foods, a category that includes all the more popular fruits and vegetables, it is generally unobtrusive and often wholly absent.

Fortunately, however, a sensitive nose is not the sole defense against an attack of botulism. Since 1895, when the isolation of *Clostridium botulinum* by the Belgian bacteriologist Emilie P. van Ermengem made possible a thorough anatomization of the disease, other, and more dependable, weapons have been worked out. One is an efficient antitoxin serum. Another is heat. Fifteen minutes of boiling (or its thermal equivalent) will destroy any number of adult *Clostridium botulinum* or any quantity of toxin. The spores are less lightly insulated. The amount of heat ordinarily required in the preliminary processing of most preserved foods has no effect whatever on them, and some have been known to survive immersion in boiling water for as long as six hours. Nevertheless, they, too, have their limitations. Even the toughest, as the food industry has been gratefully aware for almost a generation, are bound to perish if subjected for eight or ten minutes to a blast of steam under fifteen pounds of pressure. The discovery of this engaging frailty, by an international army of public and private investigators, has gradually led to the total elimination of commercially processed food as a possible source of botulism. The last outbreak in Europe involving a commercial packer occurred in 1922, in England. In the United States, the last outbreak was recorded in 1925. All subsequent cases, including, as it turned out, that of Charles Pappone, have been traced to canned, smoked, or otherwise hermetically sealed foods imperfectly processed at home.

It was close to eleven o'clock when the attending physician at the Albany Hospital made his unhappy discovery and his hopeful request that late November morning in 1949. Some twelve hours later, Dr. Morris Greenberg, director of the Bureau of Preventable Diseases of the New York City Department of Health, was roused from a bedtime doze in the living room of his home, on the upper West Side, by a telephone call. The caller was Dr. Robert F. Korns, director of the Bureau of Epidemiology and Communicable Disease Control of the State Health Department, in Albany. He was calling from his office.

"I was a little startled," Dr. Greenberg says. "I knew Korns, of course. We work together all the time. But I don't remember that he had ever called me at home before — certainly not at night. Also, for a moment I was a little baffled. I was still half asleep and Korns was pretty agitated, and about all I got was that they had found a case of botulism. That was interesting enough. It was even fascinating. Botulism is almost as rare as they come these days. I doubt if there are fifteen outbreaks a year in the entire country. To the average doctor, it's strictly a textbook disease. But Pappone was at Albany Hospital, I gathered, and he lived way upstate, in Craryville. I couldn't quite see at first where we came into the picture. When I finally did — well, I found it very hard to believe. The story — as far as it went — was this. Korns first heard of the case around three o'clock that afternoon, by way of a memo from the state laboratory. They had received a request from Albany Hospital for a quantity of botulinus antitoxin, and thought he ought to know. So did Korns. One of his epidemiologists hopped right over to the hospital. It was several hours, though, before he learned anything about the possible source of the outbreak that wasn't down on the record. Pappone, of course, couldn't talk, and his wife and daughter had just left. Neither of the two, he was told, showed any signs of illness. As a matter of routine, however, both had been given a prophylactic shot of serum. They were expected back that evening. The next report Korns received came a few minutes before he called me. His investigator had finally seen the wife and daughter, but that was about all. They were both half crazy with worry and couldn't add much to what he already knew. Or suspected. Everything seemed to point to that Thanksgiving dinner. Which meant New York City. The Bronx, to be more specific. That's where Mrs. Pappone's parents lived — the Gaglionos, I'll call them. Altogether, there were twelve of them at the dinner — all family and, except for the Pappones, all members of the household.

"Well, as I say, it looked as if the dinner was our lead. It was all there was. According to the evidence, breakfast was out. It consisted of eggs, toast, and coffee. In other words, no possible vehicle. The same went for supper. The only trouble was the whole thing sounded unlikely. Botulism doesn't happen very often in a city like New York. Or any other. City people don't can or preserve, or very seldom. You find botulism where you find big gardens — in the country and the small towns. Then, there was the dinner itself. To the best of Mrs. Pappone's recollection, everything served was fresh. Her father usually insisted on it. He was a retired chef, she said, and didn't care for canned food. But we couldn't take her word for that. Recollection isn't fact. We had to make sure.

"When Korns hung up, I got to work. I called the Gagliono home. A woman answered the phone. I introduced myself, apologized for calling so late, and asked to speak to Mr. Gagliono. She gave a kind of gasp. Then she said something — I don't know what. It was mostly Italian. And before I could reply, she was gone. I heard voices, and people moving around. It was all very strange. Presently, a man came to the phone. He sounded puzzled, but that was only natural. I started all over again. I got as far as my name and the Health Department, and then he cut in. He understood me. But he wasn't Mr. Gagliono. Mr. Gagliono was ill. Very ill. He had just suffered a serious heart attack. I was talking to the family physician. What was this all about? I told him. Although, I must admit, not quite as matter-of-factly as that. You might say that for a moment we simply stared at each other. He listened, and he asked some questions, and it was obvious that he was extremely interested. It was even more obvious, though, that he thought we were on completely the wrong track. Especially when I suggested that botulism might be a factor in his patient's trouble. He had never seen a case of botulism, he said, but he was pretty well acquainted with heart disease. The old man — he was seventy-six, I found — had had a heart condition for years. Moreover, he added, if it was botulism, wasn't it a little odd that Mr. Gagliono was the only one it hit? Because everybody else in the house was well — all eight of them. Well, I said, perhaps. Possibly. But botulism is notoriously slow. It sometimes takes five or six days for it to get a real purchase. However, at this point that wasn't the problem. The problem was the old man. He *was* sick. And the circumstances were, at least, suspicious. Sufficiently so to justify an injection of antitoxin. At once. Naturally, the doctor agreed. The only question was where to get the serum. My idea was to call my office. I knew I could get all we needed there. He suggested Fordham Hospital. It was just around the corner. If Fordham couldn't help him, he'd let me know. That was about eleven-thirty. Then I waited. I waited until midnight. No call. It looked as if Fordham had come through. So I went to bed.

"The next morning — Tuesday, November 29th — I had a word with the Commissioner, and we decided upon a formal investigation. An inspector named Schoenholtz got the assignment. I told him what we knew and what we suspected and what we had done. Then he took off for the Bronx. Before settling down to the regular routine, I put in a call to Korns and brought him up to date. That didn't take long. Neither did Korns' contribution. All he had was a progress report from Albany Hospital. Pappone was still hanging on. An hour or so later, I heard from Schoenholtz. He was up at Fordham. I can hardly say the news he had was good. And yet in a way it was — at least by implication. The facts, however, were pretty grim. Gagliono was dead. He had died in Fordham Hospital at nine-forty-five that morning. The doctor was in no way at fault. He had done everything possible. As I had assumed, he'd found some serum. It arrived a little past twelve. But the old man wouldn't take it. He didn't believe in injections. Then the doctor arranged to have him admitted to the hospital. He thought he might have better luck with him there. But the old man wouldn't go. He didn't trust hospitals. And so it went — until early morning, when the old man started sinking fast. Then the doctor became adamant. But by the time they reached the hospital, it was too late. Actually, Schoenholtz said, it had probably been too late for quite a while. There wasn't any doubt about the immediate cause of death. His heart gave out. But the chances were that even if his heart had held up, it wouldn't have made much difference. During his last few hours, it seemed, the old man had begun to develop a whole new set of symptoms. One was particularly pronounced, and significant. That was diplopia, or double vision. Well, diplopia can be indicative of various disorders, but not in this instance. In view of what we already knew, it almost had to mean botulism.

"It also meant that we were beginning to get somewhere. It fixed the occasion — pretty definitely. The only possible link between Pappone's case and his father-in-law's was that Thanksgiving dinner. Until the family reunion, they hadn't met for weeks. It was either that or the wildest of wild coincidences. All we needed now was the source of infection. That was all, but, of course, it was vital. Everything hinged on it. Including, quite conceivably, the lives of several people. Until we could turn up at least a probable vehicle, we would still be working entirely on conjecture.

"Not that I had to spell that out for Schoenholtz. Hardly. He was headed for the Gagliono home when he called in. He must have run all the way. Because I heard from him again in less than an hour. More bad news. We had another victim. She was the Gaglionos' eldest daughter, an unmarried woman of fifty. Her name, I'll say, was Rose. The clinical picture was painfully clear — prostration, diplopia, and a progressive difficulty in talking and swallowing. Schoenholtz wasn't too worried, though. The onset, as well as he could make out, had occurred around five or six that morning, and with botulism, as with a good many other diseases, the later the start, the milder the course. The family doctor had administered antitoxin, and Schoenholtz was arranging with him to have her sent over to Fordham. And, just in case, they were immunizing all the rest of the family. Schoenholtz hadn't got very far on the dinner. The place was a madhouse. But he had finally managed to pin Mrs. Gagliono down and she had given him a tentative menu. He read it off to me — chicken soup, roast turkey, mushrooms, turnips, sweet potatoes, fruit, and coffee. Nothing canned. Not even the soup. I'm bound to say my heart sank. It could hardly have been less promising. However, I told Schoenholtz to keep after Mrs. Gagliono. Maybe she had forgotten something. That looked like our only hope.

"I didn't hear from Schoenholtz again until late afternoon. Fortunately, I had plenty to do. Even so, it was a long wait. And the longer it lasted, the uneasier I got. But the minute I heard his voice, I relaxed. It had that certain sound. I knew it was all over, and it was. He hadn't just discovered the source of the trouble. He even had a sample of the vehicle. They hadn't eaten it all, and what was left went into the refrigerator with the rest of the leftovers. There were still some formalities, of course. We had to wait a few days for an ironclad confirmation from the laboratory, but that was no hardship. It was almost a hundred per cent predictable. And while we were waiting, the rest of the picture brightened. By the time we had the laboratory report, Pappone, though still very ill, was out of danger and Rose was as good as well. She had, as expected, a fairly light attack, but the antitoxin was the thing that counted. So the real credit goes to Korns. His quick hunch on the dinner probably saved her life. I can't take much credit for anything. At any rate, I was wrong about Mrs. Gagliono and the menu. She hadn't forgotten a thing. The menu was just what she said. Only, the mushrooms weren't exactly fresh.

Not to Schoenholtz's way of thinking. It was a matter of definition. She called them fresh because they didn't come out of a can. They had been bought fresh, from the corner store. But that was a couple of weeks before Thanksgiving. They ended up on the table marinated.

"Actually, Mrs. Gagliono had nothing to do with it. No more than the store. Or the grower. They were ordinary cultivated mushrooms of standard edible variety. Marinated mushrooms happened to be one of her husband's specialties. He bought them himself and he himself did all the preparing. Schoenholtz had even got hold of the recipe. It read, 'Wash in cold water. Boil in white wine for thirty minutes, and drain. Place in Mason jar, flavor with pepper and cloves, and cover with olive oil. Seal tightly.' In other words, nothing that could cause any lurking *C. botulinum* spores a moment of discomfort. And everything to encourage their growth. But the mushrooms could still have been made perfectly safe. A few minutes of heat before serving would have completely destroyed the toxin. However, that wasn't the old man's way. The jar went straight from the pantry shelf to the table.

"There was only one thing that momentarily stopped me. It was along the same lines as the question the family physician had asked. Why were there just three cases? The obvious answer, and the one Schoenholtz got, was that nobody ate any mushrooms but the old man and Pappone and Rose. The rest of them simply didn't like marinated mushrooms. There couldn't be any other explanation. Because there was nothing unusual about the mushrooms. I saw them myself. They looked good and they smelled good. Delicious, in fact. It gave me kind of a chill."

The Fog

THE Monongahela River rises in the middle Alleghenies and seeps for a hundred and twenty-eight miles through the iron and bituminous-coal fields of northeastern West Virginia and southwestern Pennsylvania to Pittsburgh. There, joining the Allegheny River, it becomes the wild Ohio. It is the only river of any consequence in the United States that flows due north, and it is also the shortest. Its course is cramped and crooked, and flanked by bluffs and precipitous hills. Within living memory, its waters were quick and green, but they are murky now with pollution, and a series of locks and dams steady its once tumultuous descent, rendering it navigable from source to mouth. Traffic on the Monongahela is heavy. Its shipping, which consists almost wholly of coal barges pushed by wheezy, coal-burning sternwheelers, exceeds in tonnage that of the Panama Canal. The river is densely industrialized. There are trucking highways along its narrow banks and interurban lincs and branches of the Pennsylvania Railroad and the New York Central and smelters and steel plants and chemical works and glass factories and foundries and coke plants and machine shops and zinc mills, and its hills and bluffs are scaled by numerous blackened mill towns. The blackest of them is the borough of Donora, in Washington County, Pennsylvania.

Donora is twenty-eight miles south of Pittsburgh and covers the tip of a lumpy point formed by the most convulsive of the Monongahela's many horseshoe bends. Though accessible by road, rail, and river, it is an extraordinarily secluded place. The river and the bluffs that lift abruptly from the water's edge to a height of four hundred and fifty feet enclose it on the north and east and south, and just above it to the west is a range of rolling but even higher hills. On its outskirts are acres of sidings and rusting gondolas, abandoned mines, smoldering slag piles, and gulches filled with rubbish. Its limits are marked by sooty signs that read, "Donora. Next to Yours the Best Town in the U.S.A." It is a harsh, gritty town, founded in 1901 and old for its age, with a gaudy main street and a thousand identical gaunt gray houses. Some of its streets are paved with concrete and some are cobbled, but many are of dirt and crushed coal. At least half of them are as steep as roofs, and several have steps instead of sidewalks. It is treeless and all but grassless, and much of it is slowly sliding downhill. After a rain, it is a smear of mud. Its vacant lots and many of its yards are mortally gullied, and one of its three cemeteries is an eroded ruin of gravelly clay and toppled tombstones. Its population is 12,300. Two-thirds of its men, and a substantial number of its women, work in its mills. There are three of them — a steel plant, a wire plant, and a zinc-and-sulphuric-acid plant — all of which are operated by the American Steel & Wire Co., a subsidiary of the United States Steel Corporation, and they line its river front for three miles. They are huge mills. Some of the buildings are two blocks long, many are five or six stories high, and all of them bristle with hundred-foot stacks perpetually plumed with black or red or sulphurous yellow smoke.

Donora is abnormally smoky. Its mills are no bigger or smokier than many, but their smoke, and the smoke from the passing boats and trains, tends to linger there. Because of the crowding bluffs and sheltering hills, there is seldom a wind, and only occasionally a breeze, to dispel it. On still days, unless the skies are high and buoyantly clear, the lower streets are always dim and there is frequently a haze on the heights. Autumn is the smokiest season. The weather is close and dull then, and there are persistent fogs as well. The densest ones generally come in October. They are greasy, gagging fogs, often intact even at high noon, and they sometimes last for two or three days. A few have lasted as long as four. One, toward the end of October, 1948, hung on for six. Unlike its predecessors, it turned out to be of considerably more than local interest. It was the second smoke-contaminated fog in history ever to reach a toxic density. The first such fog occurred in Belgium, in an industrialized stretch of the Meuse Valley, in 1930. During it several hundred people were prostrated, sixty of them fatally. The Donora fog struck down nearly six thousand. Twenty of them — five women and fifteen men — died. Nobody knows exactly what killed them, or why the others survived. At the time, not many of the stricken expected to.

The fog closed over Donora on the morning of Tuesday, October 26th. The weather was raw, cloudy, and dead calm, and it stayed that way as the fog piled up all that day and the next. By Thursday, it had stiffened adhesively into a motionless clot of smoke. That afternoon, it was just possible to see across the street, and, except for the stacks, the mills had vanished. The air began to have a sickening smell, almost a taste. It was the bittersweet reek of sulphur dioxide. Everyone who was out that day remarked on it, but no one was much concerned. The smell of sulphur dioxide, a scratchy gas given off by burning coal and melting ore, is a normal concomitant of any durable fog in Donora. This time, it merely seemed more penetrating than usual.

At about eight-thirty on Friday morning, one of Donora's eight physicians, Dr. Ralph W. Koehler, a tense, stocky man of forty-eight, stepped to his bathroom window for a look at the weather. It was, at best, unchanged. He could see nothing but a watery waste of rooftops islanded in fog. As he was turning away, a shimmer of movement in the distance caught his eye. It was a freight train creeping along the riverbank just south of town, and the sight of it shook him. He had never seen anything quite like it before. "It was the smoke," he says. "They were firing up for the grade and the smoke was belching out, but it didn't rise. I mean it didn't go up at all. It just spilled out over the lip of the stack like a black liquid, like ink or oil, and rolled down to the ground and lay there. My God, it just lay there! I thought, Well, God damn — and they talk about needing smoke control up in Pittsburgh! I've got a heart condition, and I was so disgusted my heart began to act up a little. I had to sit down on the edge of the tub and rest a minute."

Dr. Koehler and an associate, Dr. Edward Roth, who is big, heavyset, and in his middle forties, share an office on the second floor of a brownstone building one block up from the mills, on McKean Avenue, the town's main street. They have one employee, a young woman named Helen Stack, in whom are combined an attractive receptionist, an efficient secretary, and a capable nurse. Miss Stack was the first to reach the office that morning. Like Dr. Koehler and many other Donorans, she was in uncertain spirits. The fog was beginning to get on her nerves, and she had awakened with a sore throat and a cough and supposed that she was coming down with a cold. The appearance of the office deepened her depression. Everything in it was smeared with a kind of dust. "It wasn't just ordinary soot and grit," she says. "There was something white and scummy mixed up in it. It was just wet ash from the mills, but I didn't know that then. I almost hated to touch it, it was so nasty-looking. But it had to be cleaned up, so I got out a cloth and went to work." When Miss Stack had finished, she lighted a cigarette and sat down at her desk to go through the mail. It struck her that the cigarette had a very peculiar taste. She held it up and sniffed at the smoke. Then she raised it to her lips, took another puff, and doubled up in a paroxysm of coughing. For an instant, she thought she was going to be sick. "I'll never forget that taste," she says. "Oh, it was awful! It was sweet and horrible, like something rotten. It tasted the way the fog smelled, only ten times worse. I got rid of the cigarette as fast as I could and drank a glass of water, and then I felt better. What puzzled me was I'd smoked a cigarette at home after breakfast and it had tasted all right. I didn't know what to think, except that maybe it was because the fog wasn't quite as bad up the hill as here downstreet. I guess I thought my cold was probably partly to blame. I wasn't really uneasy. The big Halloween parade the Chamber of Commerce puts on every year was to be held that night, and I could hear the workmen down in the street putting up the decorations. I knew the committee wouldn't be going ahead with the parade if they thought anything was wrong. So I went on with my work, and pretty soon the Doctors came in from their early calls and it was just like any other morning."

The office hours of Dr. Koehler and Dr. Roth are the

same, from one to three in the afternoon and from seven to nine at night. Whenever possible in the afternoon, Dr. Koehler leaves promptly at three. Because of his unsteady heart, he finds it desirable to rest for a time before dinner. That Friday afternoon, he was just getting into his coat when Miss Stack announced a patient. "He was wheezing and gasping for air," Dr. Koehler says, "but there wasn't anything very surprising about that. He was one of our regular asthmatics, and the fog gets them every time. The only surprising thing was that he hadn't come in sooner. The fact is, none of our asthmatics had been in all week. Well, I did what I could for him. I gave him a shot of adrenalin or aminophyllin — some anti-spasmodic — to dilate the bronchia, so he could breathe more easily, and sent him home. I followed him out. I didn't feel so good myself."

Half an hour after Dr. Koehler left, another gasping asthmatic, an elderly steelworker, tottered into the office. "He was pretty wobbly," Miss Stack says. "Dr. Roth was still in his office, and saw him right away. I guess he wasn't much better when he came out, because I remember thinking, Poor fellow. There's nothing sadder than an asthmatic when the fog is bad. Well, he had hardly gone out the door when I heard a terrible commotion. I thought, Oh, my gosh, he's fallen down the stairs! Then there was an awful yell. I jumped up and dashed out into the hall. There was a man I'd never seen before sort of draped over the banister. He was kicking at the wall and pulling at the banister and moaning and choking and yelling at the top of his voice, 'Help! Help me! I'm dying!' I just stood there. I was petrified. Then Dr. Brown, across the hall, came running out, and he and somebody else helped the man on up the stairs and into his office. Just then, my phone began to ring. I almost bumped into Dr. Roth. He was coming out to see what was going on. When I picked up the phone, it was just like hearing that man in the hall again. It was somebody saying somebody was dying. I said Dr. Roth would be right over, but before I could even tell him, the phone started ringing again. And the minute I hung up the receiver, it rang again. That was the beginning of a terrible night. From that minute on, the phone never stopped ringing. That's the honest truth. And they were all alike. Everybody who called up said the same thing. Pain in the abdomen. Splitting headache. Nausea and vomiting. Choking and couldn't get their breath. Coughing up blood. But as soon as I got over my surprise, I calmed down. Hysterical people always end up by making me feel calm. Anyway, I managed to make a list of the first few calls and gave it to Dr. Roth. He was standing there with his hat and coat on and his bag in his hand and chewing on his cigar, and he took the list and shook his head and went out. Then I called Dr. Koehler, but his line was busy. I don't remember much about the next hour. All I know is I kept trying to reach Dr. Koehler and my phone kept ringing and my list of calls kept getting longer and longer."

One of the calls that lengthened Miss Stack's list was a summons to the home of August Z. Chambon, the burgess, or mayor, of Donora. The patient was the Burgess's mother, a widow of seventy-four, who lives with her son and his wife. "Mother Chambon was home alone that afternoon," her daughter-in-law says. "August was in Pittsburgh on business and I'd gone downstreet to do some shopping. It took me forever, the fog was so bad. Even the inside of the stores was smoky. So I didn't get home until around five-thirty. Well, I opened the door and stepped into the hall, and there was Mother Chambon. She was lying on the floor, with her coat on and a bag of cookies spilled all over beside her. Her face was blue, and she was just gasping for breath and in terrible pain. She told me she'd gone around the corner to the bakery a few minutes before, and on the way back the fog had got her. She said she barely made it to the house. Mother Chambon has bronchial trouble, but I'd never seen her so bad before. Oh, I was frightened! I helped her up — I don't know how I ever did it — and got her into bed. Then I called the doctor. It took me a long time to reach his office, and then he wasn't in. He was out making calls. I was afraid to wait until he could get here — Mother Chambon was so bad, and at her age and all — so I called another doctor. He was out, too. Finally, I got hold of Dr. Levin and he said he'd come right over, and he finally did. He gave her an injection that made her breathe easier and something to put her to sleep. She slept for sixteen solid hours. But before Dr. Levin left, I told him that there seemed to be an awful lot of sickness going on all of a sudden. I was coughing a little myself. I asked him what was happening. 'I don't know,' he said. 'Something's coming off, but I don't know what.' "

Dr. Roth returned to his office at a little past six to replenish his supply of drugs. By then, he, like Dr. Levin, was aware that something was coming off. "I knew that whatever it was we were up against was serious," he says. "I'd seen some very pitiful cases, and they weren't all asthmatics or chronics of any kind. Some were people who had never been bothered by fog before. I was worried, but I wasn't bewildered. It was no mystery. It was obvious — all the symptoms pointed to it — that the fog and smoke were to blame. I didn't think any further than that. As a matter of fact, I didn't have time to think or wonder. I was too damn busy. My biggest problem was just getting around. It was almost impossible to drive. I even had trouble finding the office. McKean Avenue was solid coal smoke. I could taste the soot when I got out of the car, and my chest felt tight. On the way up the stairs, I started coughing and I couldn't stop. I kept coughing and choking until my stomach turned over. Fortunately, Helen was out getting something to eat — I just made it to the office and into the lavatory in time. My God, I was sick! After a while, I dragged myself into my office and gave myself an injection of adrenalin and lay back in a chair. I began to feel better. I felt so much better I got out a cigar and lighted up. That practically finished me. I took one pull, and went into another paroxysm of coughing. I probably should have known better — cigars had tasted terrible all day — but I hadn't had that reaction before. Then I heard the phone ringing. I guess it must have been ringing off and on all along. I thought about answering it, but I didn't have the strength to move. I just lay there in my chair and let it ring."

When Miss Stack came into the office a few minutes later, the telephone was still ringing. She had answered it and added the call to her list before she realized that she was not alone. "I heard someone groaning," she says. "Dr. Roth's door was open and I looked in. I almost jumped, I was so startled. He was slumped down in his chair, and his face was brick red and dripping with perspiration. I wanted to help him, but he said there wasn't anything to do. He told me what had happened. 'I'm all right now,' he said. 'I'll get going again in a minute. You go ahead and answer the phone.' It was ringing again. The next thing I knew, the office was full of patients, all of them coughing and groaning. I was about ready to break down and cry. I had talked to Dr. Koehler by that time and he knew what was happening. He had been out on calls from home. 'I'm coughing and sick myself,' he said, 'but I'll go out again as soon as I can.' I tried to keep calm, but with both Doctors sick and the office full of patients and the phone ringing, I just didn't know which way to turn. Dr. Roth saw two or three of the worst patients. Oh, he looked ghastly! He really looked worse than some of the patients. Finally, he said he couldn't see any more, that the emergency house calls had to come first, and grabbed up his stuff and went out. The office was still full of patients, and I went around explaining things to them. It was awful. There wasn't anything to do but close up, but I've never felt so heartless. Some of them were so sick and miserable. And right in the middle of everything the parade came marching down the street. People were cheering and yelling, and the bands were playing. I could hardly believe my ears. It just didn't seem possible."

The sounds of revelry that reached Miss Stack were deceptive. The parade, though well attended, was not an unqualified success. "I went out for a few minutes and watched it," the younger Mrs. Chambon says. "It went right by our house. August wasn't home yet, and after what had happened to Mother Chambon, I thought it might cheer me up a little. It did and it didn't. Everybody was talking about the fog and wondering when it would end, and some of them had heard there was sickness, but nobody seemed at all worried. As far as I could tell, all the sick people were old. That made things look not too bad. The fog always affects the old people. But as far as the parade was concerned, it was a waste of time. You really couldn't see a thing. They were just like shadows marching by. It was kind of uncanny. Especially since most of the people in the crowd had handkerchiefs tied over their nose and mouth to keep out the smoke. All the children did. But, even so, everybody was coughing. I was glad to get back in the house. I guess everybody was. The minute it was over, everybody scattered. They just vanished. In two minutes there wasn't a soul left on the street. It was as quiet as midnight."

Among the several organizations that participated in the parade was the Donora Fire Department. The force consists of about thirty volunteers and two full-time men. The latter, who live at the firehouse, are the chief, John Volk, a wiry man in his fifties, and his assistant and driver, a hard, round-faced young man named Russell Davis. Immediately after the parade, they returned to the firehouse. "As a rule," Chief Volk says, "I like a parade. "We've got some nice equipment here, and I don't mind showing it off. But I didn't get much pleasure out of that one. Nobody could see us, hardly, and we couldn't see them. That fog was black as a derby hat. It had us all coughing. It was a relief to head for home. We hadn't much more than got back to the station, though, and got the trucks put away and said good night to the fellows than the phone rang. Russ and I were just sitting down to drink some coffee. I dreaded to answer it. On a night like that, a fire could have been real mean. But it wasn't any fire. It was a fellow up the street, and the fog had got him. He said he was choking to death and couldn't get a doctor, and what he wanted was our inhalator. He needed air. Russ says I just stood there with my mouth hanging open. I don't remember what I thought. I guess I was trying to think what to do as much as anything else. I didn't disbelieve him — he sounded half dead already — but, naturally, we're not supposed to go running around treating the sick. But what the hell, you can't let a man die! So I told him O.K. I told Russ to take the car and go. The way it turned out, I figure we did the right thing. I've never heard anybody say different."

"That guy was only the first," Davis says. "From then on, it was one emergency call after another. I didn't get to bed until Sunday. Neither did John. I don't know how many calls we had, but I do know this: We had around eight hundred cubic feet of oxygen on hand when I started out Friday night, and we ended up by borrowing from McKeesport and Monessen and Monongahela and Charleroi and everywhere around here. I never want to go through a thing like that again. I was laid up for a week after. There never was such a fog. You couldn't see your hand in front of your face, day or night. Hell, even inside the station the air was blue. I drove on the left side of the street with my head out the window, steering by scraping the curb. We've had bad fogs here before. A guy lost his car in one. He'd come to a fork in the road and didn't know where he was, and got out to try and tell which way to go. When he turned back to his car, he couldn't find it. He had no idea where it was until, finally, he stopped and listened and heard the engine. That guided him back. Well, by God, this fog was so bad you couldn't even get a car to idle. I'd take my foot off the accelerator and — bango! — the engine would stall. There just wasn't any oxygen in the air. I don't know how I kept breathing. I don't know how anybody did. I found people laying in bed and laying on the floor. Some of them were laying there and they didn't give a damn whether they died or not. I found some down in the basement with the furnace draft open and their head stuck inside, trying to get air that way. What I did when I got to a place was throw a sheet or a blanket over the patient and stick a cylinder of oxygen underneath and crack the valves for fifteen minutes or so. By God, that rallied them! I didn't take any myself. What I did every time I came back to the station was have a little shot of whiskey. That seemed to help. It eased my throat. There was one funny thing about the whole thing. Nobody seemed to realize what was going on. Everybody seemed to think he was the only sick man in town. I don't know what they figured was keeping the doctors so busy. I guess everybody was so miserable they just didn't think."

Toward midnight, Dr. Roth abandoned his car and continued his rounds on foot. He found not only that walking was less of a strain but that he made better time. He walked the streets all night, but he was seldom lonely. Often, as he entered or left a house, he encountered a colleague. "We all had practically the same calls," Dr. M. J. Hannigan, the president of the Donora Medical Association, says. "Some people called every doctor in town. It was pretty discouraging to finally get someplace and drag yourself up the steps and then be told that Dr. So-and-So had just been there. Not that I blame them, though. Far from it. There were a couple of times when I was about ready to call for help myself. Frankly, I don't know how any of us doctors managed to hold out and keep going that night."

Not all of them did. Dr. Koehler made his last call that night at one o'clock. "I had to go home," he says. "God knows I didn't want to. I'd hardly made a dent in my list. Every time I called home or the Physicians' Exchange, it doubled. But my heart gave out. I couldn't go on any longer without some rest. The last thing I heard as I got into bed was my wife answering the phone. And the phone was the first thing I heard in the morning. It was as though I hadn't been to sleep at all." While Dr. Koehler was bolting a cup of coffee, the telephone rang again. This time, it was Miss Stack. They conferred briefly about the patients he had seen during the night and those he planned to see that morning. Among the latter was a sixty-four-year-old steelworker named Ignatz Hollowitti. "One of the Hollowitti girls, Dorothy, is a good friend of mine," Miss Stack says. "So as soon as I finished talking to Dr. Koehler, I called her to tell her that Doctor would be right over. I wanted to relieve her mind. Dorothy was crying when she answered the phone. I'll never forget what she said. She said, 'Oh, Helen — my dad just died! He's dead!' I don't remember what I said. I was simply stunned. I suppose I said what people say. I must have. But all I could think was, My gosh, if people are dying — why, this is tragic! Nothing like this has ever happened before!"

Mr. Hollowitti was not the first victim of the fog. He was the sixth. The first was a retired steelworker of seventy named Ivan Ceh. According to the records of the undertaker who was called in — Rudolph Schwerha, whose establishment is the largest in Donora — Mr. Ceh died at one-thirty Saturday morning. "I was notified at two," Mr. Schwerha says. "There is a note to such effect in my book. I thought nothing, of course. The call awakened me from sleep, but in my profession anything is to be expected. I reassured the bereaved and called my driver and sent him for the body. He was gone forever. The fog that night was impossible. It was a neighborhood case — only two blocks to go, and my driver works quick — but it was thirty minutes by the clock before I heard the service car in the drive. At that moment, again the phone rang. Another case. Now I was surprised. Two different cases so soon together in this size town doesn't happen every day. But there was no time then for thinking.

There was work to do. I must go with my driver for the second body. It was in the Sunnyside section, north of town, too far in such weather for one man alone. The fog, when we got down by the mills, was unbelievable. Nothing could be seen. It was like a blanket. Our fog lights were useless, and even with the fog spotlight on, the white line in the street was invisible. I began to worry. What if we should bump a parked car? What if we should fall off the road? Finally, I told my driver, 'Stop! I'll take the wheel. You walk in front and show the way.' So we did that for two miles. Then we were in the country. I know that section like my hand, but we had missed the house. So we had to turn around and go back. That was an awful time. We were on the side of a hill, with a terrible drop on one side and no fence. I was afraid every minute. But we made it, moving by inches, and pretty soon I found the house. The case was an old man and he had died all of a sudden. Acute cardiac dilation. When we were ready, we started back. Then I began to feel sick. The fog was getting me. There was an awful tickle in my throat. I was coughing and ready to vomit. I called to my driver that I had to stop and get out. He was ready to stop, I guess. Already he had walked four or five miles. But I envied him. He was well and I was awful sick. I leaned against the car, coughing and gagging, and at last I riffled a few times. Then I was much better. I could drive. So we went on, and finally we were home. My wife was standing at the door. Before she spoke, I knew what she would say. I thought, Oh, my God — another! I knew it by her face. And after that came another. Then another. There seemed to be no end. By ten o'clock in the morning, I had nine bodies waiting here. Then I heard that DeRienzo and Lawson, the other morticians, each had one. Eleven people dead! My driver and I kept looking at each other. What was happening? We didn't know. I thought probably the fog was the reason. It had the smell of poison. But we didn't know."

Mr. Schwerha's bewilderment was not widely shared. Most Donorans were still unaware Saturday morning that anything was happening. They had no way of knowing. Donora has no radio station, and its one newspaper, the *Herald-American*, is published only five days a week, Monday through Friday. It was past noon before a rumor of widespread illness began to drift through town. The news reached August Chambon at about two o'clock. In addition to being burgess, an office that is more an honor than a livelihood, Mr. Chambon operates a moving-and-storage business, and he had been out of town on a job all morning. "There was a message waiting for me when I got home," he says. "John Elco, of the Legion, had called and wanted me at the Borough Building right away. I wondered what the hell, but I went right over. It isn't like John to get excited over nothing. The fog didn't even enter my mind. Of course, I'd heard there were some people sick from it. My wife had told me that. But I hadn't paid it any special significance. I just thought they were like Mother — old people that were always bothered by fog. Jesus, in a town like this you've got to expect fog. It's natural. At least, that's what I thought then. So I was astonished when John told me that the fog was causing sickness all over town. I was just about floored. That's a fact. Because I felt fine myself. I was hardly even coughing much. Well, as soon as I'd talked to John and the other fellows he had rounded up, I started in to do what I could. Something had already been done. John and Cora Vernon, the Red Cross director, were setting up an emergency-aid station in the Community Center. We don't have a hospital here. The nearest one is at Charleroi. Mrs. Vernon was getting a doctor she knew there to come over and take charge of the station, and the Legion was arranging for cars and volunteer nurses. The idea was to get a little organization in things — everything was confused as hell — and also to give our doctors a rest. They'd been working steady for thirty-six hours or more. Mrs. Vernon was fixing it so when somebody called a doctor's number, they would be switched to the Center and everything would be handled from there. I've worked in the mills and I've dug coal, but I never worked any harder than I worked that day. Or was so worried. Mostly I was on the phone. I called every town around here to send supplies for the station and oxygen for the firemen. I even called Pittsburgh. Maybe I overdid it. There was stuff pouring in here for a week. But what I wanted to be was prepared for anything. The way that fog looked that day, it wasn't ever going to lift. And then the rumors started going around that now people were dying. Oh, Jesus! Then I was scared. I heard all kinds of reports. Four dead. Ten dead. Thirteen dead. I did the only thing I could think of. I notified the State Health Department, and I called a special meeting of the Council and our Board of Health and the mill officials for the first thing Sunday morning. I wanted to have it right then, but I couldn't get hold of everybody — it was Saturday night. Every time I looked up from the phone, I'd hear a new rumor. Usually a bigger one. I guess I heard everything but the truth. What I was really afraid of was that they might set off a panic. That's what I kept dreading. I needn't have worried, though. The way it turned out, half the town had hardly heard that there was anybody even sick until

Sunday night, when Walter Winchell opened his big mouth on the radio. By then, thank God, it was all over."

The emergency-aid station, generously staffed and abundantly supplied with drugs and oxygen inhalators, opened at eight o'clock Saturday night. "We were ready for anything and prepared for the worst," Mrs. Vernon says. "We even had an ambulance at our disposal. Phillip DeRienzo, the undertaker, loaned it to us. But almost nothing happened. Altogether, we brought in just eight patients. Seven, to be exact. One was dead when the car arrived. Three were very bad and we sent them to the hospital in Charleroi. The others we just treated and sent home. It was really very queer. The fog was as black and nasty as ever that night, or worse, but all of a sudden the calls for a doctor just seemed to trickle out and stop. It was as though everybody was sick who was going to be sick. I don't believe we had a call after midnight. I knew then that we'd seen the worst of it."

Dr. Roth had reached that conclusion, though on more slender evidence, several hours before. "I'd had a call about noon from a woman who said two men roomers in her house were in bad shape," he says. "It was nine or nine-thirty by the time I finally got around to seeing them. Only, I never saw them. The landlady yelled up to them that I was there, and they yelled right back, "Tell him never mind. We're O.K. now.' Well, that was good enough for me. I decided things must be letting up. I picked up my grip and walked home and fell into bed. I was dead-beat."

There was no visible indication that the fog was beginning to relax its smothering grip when the group summoned by Burgess Chambon assembled at the Borough Building the next morning to discuss the calamity. It was another soggy, silent, midnight day. "That morning was the worst," the Burgess says. "It wasn't just that the fog was still hanging on. We'd begun to get some true facts. We didn't have any real idea how many people were sick. That didn't come out for months. We thought a few hundred. But we did have the number of deaths. It took the heart out of you. The rumors hadn't come close to it. It was eighteen. I guess we talked about that first. Then the question of the mills came up. The smoke. L. J. Westhaver, who was general superintendent of the steel and wire works then, was there, and so was the head of the zinc plant, M. M. Neale. I asked them to shut down for the duration. They said they already had. They had started banking the fires at six that morning. They went on to say, though, that they were sure the mills had nothing to do with the trouble. We didn't know what to think. Everybody was at a loss to point the finger at anything in particular. There just didn't seem to be any explanation. We had another meeting that afternoon. It was the same thing all over again. We talked and we wondered and we worried. We couldn't think of anything to do that hadn't already been done. I think we heard about the nineteenth death before we broke up. We thought for a week that was the last. Then one more finally died. I don't remember exactly what all we did or said that afternoon. What I remember is after we broke up. When we came out of the building, it was raining. Maybe it was only drizzling then — I guess the real rain didn't set in until evening — but, even so, there was a hell of a difference. The air was different. It didn't get you any more. You could breathe."

The investigation of the disaster lasted almost a year. It was not only the world's first full-blooded examination of the general problem of air pollution but one of the most exhaustive inquiries of any kind ever made in the field of public health. Its course was directed jointly by Dr. Joseph Shilen, director of the Bureau of Industrial Hygiene of the Pennsylvania Department of Health, and Dr. J. G. Townsend, chief of the Division of Industrial Hygiene of the United States Public Health Service, and at times it involved the entire technical personnel of both agencies. The Public Health Service assigned to the case nine engineers, seven physicians, six nurses, five chemists, three statisticians, two meteorologists, two dentists, and a veterinarian. The force under the immediate direction of Dr. Shilen, though necessarily somewhat smaller, was similarly composed.

The investigation followed three main lines, embracing the clinical, the environmental, and the meteorological aspects of the occurrence. Of these, the meteorological inquiry was the most nearly conclusive. It was also the most reassuring. It indicated that while the situation of Donora is unwholesomely conducive to the accumulation of smoke and fog, the immediate cause of the October, 1948, visitation was a freak of nature known to meteorologists as a temperature inversion. This phenomenon is, as its name suggests, characterized by a temporary, and usually brief, reversal of the normal atmospheric conditions, in which the air near the earth is warmer than the air higher up. Its result is a more or less complete immobilization of the convection currents in the lower air by which gases and fumes are ordinarily carried upward, away from the earth.

The clinical findings, with one or two exceptions, were more confirmatory than illuminating. One of the revelations, which was gleaned from several months of tireless interviewing, was that thousands, rather than just hundreds, had been ill during the fog. For the most part, the findings demonstrated, to the surprise of neither the investigators nor the Donora physicians, that the affection was essentially an irritation of the respiratory tract, that its severity increased in proportion to the age of the victim and his predisposition to cardio-respiratory ailments, and that the ultimate cause of death was suffocation.

The environmental study, the major phase of which was an analysis of the multiplicity of gases emitted by the mills, boats, and trains, was, in a positive sense, almost wholly unrewarding. It failed to determine the direct causative agent. Still, its results, though negative, were not without value. They showed, contrary to expectation, that no one of the several stack gases known to be irritant — among them fluoride, chloride, hydrogen sulphide, cadmium oxide, and sulphur dioxide — could have been present in the air in sufficient concentration to produce serious illness. "It seems reasonable to state," Dr. Helmuth H. Schrenk, chief of the Environmental Investigations Branch of the Public Health Service's Division of Industrial Hygiene, has written of this phase of the inquiry, "that while no single substance was responsible for the . . . episode, the syndrome could have been produced by a combination, or summation of the action, of two or more of the contaminants. Sulphur dioxide and its oxidation products, together with particulate matter [soot and fly ash], are considered significant contaminants. However, the significance of the other irritants as important adjuvants to the biological effects cannot be finally estimated on the basis of present knowledge. It is important to emphasize that information available on the toxicological effects of mixed irritant gases is meagre and data on possible enhanced action due to adsorption of gases on particulate matter is limited." To this, Dr. Leonard A. Scheele, Surgeon General of the Service, has added, "One of the most important results of the study is to show us what we do not know."

Funeral services for most of the victims of the fog were held on Tuesday, November 2nd. Monday had been a day of battering rain, but the weather cleared in the night, and Tuesday was fine. "It was like a day in spring," Mr. Schwerha says. "I think I have never seen such a beautiful blue sky or such a shining sun or such pretty white clouds. Even the trees in the cemetery seemed to have color. I kept looking up all day."